Ear, Nose, and Throat Issues in Primary Care

Editor

DONNA M. KAMINSKI

PRIMARY CARE:
CLINICS IN OFFICE PRACTICE

www.primarycare.theclinics.com

Consulting Editor
JOEL J. HEIDELBAUGH

March 2025 • Volume 52 • Number 1

ELSEVIER

1600 John F. Kennedy Boulevard • Suite 1800 • Philadelphia, Pennsylvania, 19103-2899

http://www.theclinics.com

PRIMARY CARE: CLINICS IN OFFICE PRACTICE Volume 52, Number 1
March 2025 ISSN 0095-4543, ISBN-13: 978-0-443-31646-3

Editor: Taylor Hayes
Developmental Editor: Nitesh Barthwal

Primary Care: Clinics in Office Practice (ISSN: 0095-4543) is published quarterly by Elsevier Inc., 360 Park Avenue South, New York, NY 10010-1710. Months of issue are March, June, September, and December. Periodicals postage paid at New York, NY and additional mailing offices. Subscription prices are $282.00 per year (US individuals), $100.00 (US students), $337.00 (Canadian individuals), $100.00 (Canadian students), $398.00 (international individuals), and $175.00 (international students). For institutional access pricing please contact Customer Service via the contact information below. Foreign air speed delivery is included in all *Clinics* subscription prices. All prices are subject to change without notice. Orders will be billed at individual rate until proof of status is received. Foreign air speed delivery is included in all *Clinics* subscription prices. All prices are subject to change without notice. Orders, claims, and journal inquiries: Please visit our Support Hub page https://service.elsevier.com for assistance.

Reprints. For copies of 100 or more, of articles in this publication, please contact the Commercial Reprints Department, Elsevier Inc., 360 Park Avenue South, New York, NY 10010-1710. Tel. 212-633-3874; Fax: 212-633-3820; E-mail: reprints@elsevier.com.

Primary Care: Clinics in Office Practice is covered in *MEDLINE/PubMed (Index Medicus)* and *EMBASE/ Excerpta Medica, Current Contents/Clinical Medicine,* and *ISI/BIOMED.*

Printed in the United States of America.

Contributors

CONSULTING EDITOR

JOEL J. HEIDELBAUGH, MD, FAAFP, FACG
Clinical Professor, Departments of Family Medicine and Urology, University of Michigan
Medical School, Ann Arbor, Michigan; Ypsilanti Health Center, Ypsilanti, Michigan

EDITOR

DONNA M. KAMINSKI, DO, MPH, FAAFP
Assistant Director, Department of Family Medicine, Rutgers Robert Wood Johnson
University Hospital Somerset, Somerset Family Practice Family Medicine Residency
Program, Somerville, New Jersey

AUTHORS

CLAUDIA ALVAREZ, DO
Family Medicine Residency Faculty, Sickle Cell Transition Clinic Director, Department of
Family Medicine, Harbor-UCLA Medical Center, Harbor City, California

NICHOLAS ANDERSON, MD
Director, Sleep and Insomnia Center, Hawaii Pacific Neuroscience, Honolulu, Hawaii

SIERRA ANDERSON, MD
PGY-2 Family Medicine Resident, Department of Family Medicine, Indiana University
School of Medicine, Indianapolis, Indiana

DANIEL ARRIOLA, MD
PGY-3 Resident Physician, Family Medicine Residency, Loma Linda University Medical
Center-Murrieta, Murrieta, Loma Linda University School of Medicine, Loma Linda,
California

AYSHA AZAM, DO
Clinical Faculty, Department of Family Medicine, Robert Wood Johnson University
Hospital Somerset, Somerville, New Jersey

ADITY BHATTACHARYYA, MD, FAAFP
Associate Director, JFK Family Medicine Residency Program, Edison, New Jersey;
Associate Professor, Department of Family Medicine, Hackensack Meridian School of
Medicine, Nutley, New Jersey

JENNIFER BUSTAMANTE, DO
Assistant Program Director, NSUKPCOM Family Medicine Residency Program, Family
Medicine Physician, Department of Family Medicine, Evara Health, Clearwater, Florida

JOHN CHENG, MD
Associate Clinical Professor, Department of Family Medicine, David Geffen School of Medicine at UCLA, Clinic Director, Harbor-UCLA Family Medicine Clinic, Harbor-UCLA Medical Center, Harbor City, California

SARAH N. DALRYMPLE, MD
Assistant Professor and Associate Residency Program Director, Department of Family Medicine, University of Virginia Health, Charlottesville, Virginia

JOHN D. GAZEWOOD, MD, MSPH
Associate Professor, Residency Program Director and Vice Chair, Department of Family Medicine, University of Virginia Health, Charlottesville, Virginia

JENNIFER GOODFRED, DO, FAAFP
Associate Program Director, Associate Professor, Department of Family Medicine, Baptist Memorial Hospital, Memphis, Tennessee

ROSE HALL, DO
Medical Director, Department of Family Medicine, McLaren Flint Family Medicine Residency Program, Flint, Michigan

ALLISON HOLLEY, MD
Assistant Professor, Department of Family Medicine, Florida Atlantic University College of Medicine, Boca Raton, Florida

GRETCHEN M. IRWIN, MD, MBA
Associate Professor with Tenure, Department of Family and Community Medicine, University of Kansas School of Medicine- Wichita, Wichita, Kansas

JASMINE KAUR, MD
PGY-3 Resident in Family Medicine, Department of Family Medicine, McLaren Flint Family Medicine Residency Program, Flint, Michigan

ARCHANA KUDRIMOTI, MBBS, MPH
Professor, Department of Family and Community Medicine, University of Kentucky, UK Healthcare at Turfland, Lexington, Kentucky

MAHESH R. KUDRIMOTI, MD
Radiation Oncologist, St Elizabeth Cancer Center, Greendale, Indiana

JORDAN LEATHERMAN, MD
PGY-3 Resident Physician, Department of Family and Community Medicine, University of Kansas School of Medicine- Wichita, Wichita, Kansas

DANIELA LOBO, MD
Assistant Professor of Clinical Family Medicine, Department of Family Medicine, Indiana University School of Medicine, Indianapolis, Indiana

LARRY NGO, MD, FAAP
Assistant Professor, Department of Pediatrics, Loma Linda University Children's Hospital, Loma Linda University School of Medicine, Loma Linda, California

VAN TUONG NGOC NGUYEN, DO, FAAFP, DipABOM
Associate Professor, Department of Family Medicine, Loma Linda University Health, Program Director, Family Medicine Residency, Loma Linda University Medical Center-Murrieta, Murrieta, Loma Linda University School of Medicine, Loma Linda, California

NIRALI PATEL, DO, MS
Assistant Director, JFK Family Medicine Residency Program, Edison, New Jersey; Assistant Professor, Department of Family Medicine, Hackensack Meridian School of Medicine, Nutley, New Jersey

BERNADETTE PENDERGRAPH, MD
Associate Program Director, Harbor-UCLA Family Medicine Residency Program, Program Director, Harbor-UCLA/Team to Win/Kaiser Permanente Sports Medicine Fellowship, Associate Clinical Professor, Department of Family Medicine, David Geffen School of Medicine at UCLA, Harbor City, California

MELANIE PENDERGRASS, DO
Family Medicine Specialist, Department of Family Medicine, McLaren Flint, Flint, Michigan

PARVATHI PERUMAREDDI, DO
Associate Professor of Family Medicine, Department of Medicine, Schmidt College of Medicine, Florida Atlantic University, Boca Raton, Florida

PRABHAT K. POKHREL, MS, MD, PhD, FAAFP
Program Director, Department of Family Medicine, McLaren Flint, Flint, Michigan

CARLOS R. RODRIGUEZ, MD, FAAFP
Program Director, NSU-KPCOM Family Medicine Residency Program, Director, Department of Family Medicine, Evara Health, Clearwater, Florida

JESSICA H. ROW, MD
Assistant Professor, Department of Family Medicine, University of Virginia Health, Charlottesville, Virginia

LAUREN SIMON, MD, MPH
Associate Program Director, Associate Professor, Department of Family Medicine, Baptist Memorial Hospital, Murrieta, California

SIMRAN SINGH, DO
Fellow, Sports Medicine, University of Buffalo Primary Care Sports Medicine, Buffalo, New York

ERICA STRATTON, MD
Assistant Professor, Department of Family Medicine, Loma Linda University Health, Core Faculty, Family Medicine Residency, Loma Linda University Medical Center-Murrieta, Murrieta, Loma Linda University School of Medicine, Loma Linda, California

TAJWAR TAHER, MD
Attending Physician, Department of Family Medicine, Willamette Valley Medical Center, McMinnville, Oregon

PATTY TRAN, DO
Assistant Professor, Department of Family Medicine and Community Health, John A Burns School of Medicine, University of Hawaii, Aiea, Hawaii

TONY TRAN, DO
PGY-2 Resident Physician, NSUKPCOM Family Medicine Resident, Department of Family Medicine, Evara Health, Clearwater, Florida

SARAH WIGGILL, MD, MSc
Assistant Professor, Department of Family Medicine, Florida Atlantic University College of Medicine, Boca Raton, Florida

JAMES WILCOX, MD, RMSK, FAAFP
Assistant Professor of Clinical Family Medicine, Department of Family Medicine, Indiana University School of Medicine, Indianapolis, Indiana

FRANCES WU, MD
Assistant Program Director, Family Medicine Residency Program, Department of Family Medicine, Rutgers-RWJUH Somerset, Somerville, New Jersey

Contents

primarily a clinical diagnosis which can be confirmed with specific testing as indicated to ascertain causative agents. Initial treatment includes using topical agents like intranasal corticosteroids and inhaled antihistamines as the first-line therapies for both allergic rhinitis and chronic rhinitis. Therapy can evolve in a stepwise manner depending on the primary symptom complaint prior to referral for advanced therapies such as allergen immunotherapy.

Obstructive sleep apnea (OSA) is a very common and underdiagnosed condition across the world. It affects both pediatric and adult populations in unique but important ways. Long-term health risks associated with OSA include cardiovascular conditions, metabolic disorders, depression as well as poor work performance, and increased risk of motor vehicle accidents. Accurate and precise testing is vital to ensure accurate treatment, and specific testing methods are reviewed. Treatment options are discussed in detail for both adult and pediatric populations.

Tinnitus is considered a symptom and not a diagnosis. It varies in its presentation from unilateral to bilateral and intermittent to constant. Typically, it is of unknown etiology but can be due to a secondary medical condition. Work up should include obtaining a detailed history and performing a focused physical examination as well as assessment of potential concomitant hearing loss as these often go hand in hand. Management includes helping the patient cope with their tinnitus using tools such as cognitive behavioral therapy among others. Education is also crucial to help patients understand and overcome the challenges associated with this symptom.

About 85% of US adults with hearing loss have unmet hearing needs, creating significant individual and population effects on chronic conditions, socioeconomics, and quality of life. This article reviews the diagnosis and management of hearing loss, overcoming systemic barriers, resources in limited primary care settings, and a multidisciplinary approach.

This study provides a comprehensive overview of sinusitis, detailing its pathophysiology, clinical manifestations, diagnostic criteria, and management strategies. Sinusitis, characterized by inflammation of the paranasal sinuses, can be acute, subacute, recurrent, or chronic, with distinct clinical presentations and treatment approaches. Diagnosis relies on clinical evaluation, imaging studies, and occasionally nasal endoscopy. Treatment encompasses both pharmacologic and non-pharmacological interventions, including antibiotics for bacterial cases and intranasal corticosteroids to reduce inflammation. Surgical interventions like functional endoscopic sinus surgery may be required for refractory cases. Emerging therapies, such as biologics and minimally invasive procedures, offer promising alternatives to traditional management approaches.

While pharyngitis is a common primary care complaint, evidence reveals that this diagnosis is an area where antibiotic therapy is frequently misused. Appropriate diagnosis and management of pharyngitis is crucial to ensure antimicrobial stewardship and improve patient safety and outcomes. Pharyngitis etiologies include both infectious and noninfectious sources such as bacteria, viruses, fungal organisms, trauma, irritants, laryngopharyngeal reflux, and medications. Clinicians need to obtain a thorough history and careful physical examination, along with appropriate diagnostic testing when indicated, to ensure treatment plans are targeted toward the most likely pharyngitis etiology.

Bell's palsy is acute weakness of the facial muscles associated with compression of cranial nerve VII. The annual incidence is 20 to 30 per 100,000. Diagnosis is based on a thorough history and physical examination, with careful attention to exclude other causes of facial weakness, such as stroke or Lyme disease. Oral corticosteroids improve recovery rates and antiviral medications reduce synkinesis. Most patients will recover completely. Physical therapy and Botox injections can help patients with persistent symptoms. The roles of surgery and acupuncture remain unclear. Close follow-up is warranted and patients without improvement should be referred to a specialist.

Vocal cord disorders present with a variety of symptoms including dysphonia, respiratory symptoms, and stridor. When evaluating symptoms, a complete history and through head, neck, and neurologic examinations are necessary. If dysphonia persists for greater than 4 w or there is associated smoking, then larngoscopy is necessary to evaluate the vocal folds. Empiric treatment of dysphonia is not recommended without direct visualization of the vocal folds. Most masses of the vocal folds are benign and resolve with voice hygiene and speech therapy. Surgery is reserved for persistent symptomatic nodules and cancerous lesions.

Head and neck cancers are heterogenous cancers with rising incidence of treatable/curative cancers. They are treated comprehensively by multidisciplinary teams. Survivors of head and neck cancers often deal with the sequalae of therapy and with increasing survival rates, it is anticipated that the primary care physicians are going to encounter more patients in their clinics in the coming years. The clinicians should be aware of physiologic and functional changes in vital organs involving daily activities such as eating, drinking, speech and communication, and also be prepared to be a part of the cancer survivorship plans.

Temporomandibular junction disorders (TMD) are a common problem for patients presenting to the primary care office. Symptoms may be acute or chronic. Patients may report a variety of complaints such as: painful clicking at the joint, difficulty opening the mouth or chewing, tenderness in the muscles around the joint, headaches, or tinnitus. Physical examination findings vary and may include palpable tenderness or spasm of the pterygoid muscles, palpable or audible clicking at the joint, wear and tear of tooth enamel, or dental malocclusion. Most TMDs respond well to conservative therapy, but some patients may benefit from more invasive treatments.

Dysphagia, or difficulty swallowing, has significant impacts on patients' quality of life. A thorough history and physical examination can provide important information to determine if dysphagia is originating from oropharyngeal or esophageal causes. Identifying the underlying pathology contributing to dysphagia allows for optimal treatment and improved quality of life.

PRIMARY CARE:
CLINICS IN OFFICE PRACTICE

SERIES OF RELATED INTEREST

Medical Clinics (http://www.medical.theclinics.com)
Physician Assistant Clinics (https://www.physicianassistant.theclinics.com)

THE CLINICS ARE AVAILABLE ONLINE!
Access your subscription at:
www.theclinics.com

Foreword
Spinning Days and Ringing Nights

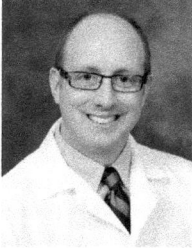

Joel J. Heidelbaugh, MD, FAAFP, FACG
Consulting Editor

A recent discussion with a medical student centered on how it is quite common for presenting concerns to overlap across multiple organ systems. Case in point was our very next patient, whose chief concern written on her intake form was actually "spinning days and ringing nights." Our patient, a 33-year-old otherwise healthy woman, presented with the progressive inability to maintain her balance, coupled with an increasingly loud ringing sensation bilaterally that prevented her from sleeping soundly on most nights. My very knowledgeable student created an extensive differential diagnosis, therapeutic plans, and a referral list that spanned neurology, neurosurgery, otolaryngology, psychiatry, and even cardiology. Now, we had the daunting task of narrowing the differential and workup, providing support to our patient, and finding the correct answers.

Disorders of the ear, nose, and throat continue to be among the most common that we encounter in primary care practices. While many are quite simple to diagnose and treat, others require detailed workups to tailor appropriate initial treatments prior to consideration of subspecialty referral. In recent years, there have been significant advances in the treatment for hearing loss, dysphonia, tinnitus, and vestibular conditions. Primary care clinicians diagnose the majority of cancers, and head and neck cancers are increasing in incidence. With significant attention toward diagnosis and treatment of obstructive sleep apnea, there are now additional training programs for primary care residency graduates to gain skills and incorporate elements of sleep medicine into their practices.

As for every issue of *Primary Care: Clinics in Office Practice*, I have many people to acknowledge for their dedicated and diligent work. Dr Donna Kaminski created the vision for an outstanding, very timely, and unique issue of articles on common ear, nose, and throat conditions encountered in primary care practices. Over 30 clinicians provided expert authorship of impactful articles highlighting the latest literature and evidence. As I should mention for each *Primary Care: Clinics in Office Practice* issue, I

Prim Care Clin Office Pract 52 (2025) xiii–xiv
https://doi.org/10.1016/j.pop.2024.12.002
0095-4543/25/© 2024 Published by Elsevier Inc.

give praise to our phenomenal editorial, leadership, and production staff at Elsevier without whom the final product that you hold would not be possible.

Joel J. Heidelbaugh, MD, FAAFP, FACG
Departments of Family Medicine
and Urology
University of Michigan Medical School
Ann Arbor, MI 48103, USA

Ypsilanti Health Center
200 Arnet, Suite 200
Ypsilanti, MI 48198, USA

E-mail address:
jheidel@umich.edu

Preface

An Emerging Need for Ear, Nose, and Throat Care in the Primary Care Setting

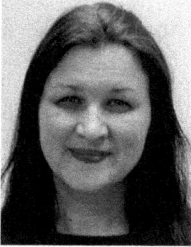

Donna M. Kaminski, DO, MPH, FAAFP
Editor

The US Department of Health and Human Services anticipates that in this year, 2025, we will have a shortage of 1620 otolaryngologists, despite an increase in the use of advance practice providers.[1] This is likely to have a deep impact on patients and on us as primary care providers, as ear, nose, and throat (ENT) concerns are quite frequent in the primary care setting. One in eight patient visits will include an ENT-related complaint. The rates are even higher in children. Up to 29% of patient visit complaints in children include an ENT complaint, which is more than three times more common than in adults.[2]

This anticipated shortage calls for an increasing need for common ENT issues to be managed by primary care clinicians. Therefore, we have designed this issue to focus on common ENT issues, such as acute and chronic middle and external otitis, vestibular disorders, tonsillitis, rhinitis, sleep apnea, tinnitus, hearing loss, sinusitis, pharyngitis, Bell palsy, vocal cord disorders, head and neck cancers, temporomandibular disorders, and swallowing disorders. Our hope is that it will serve as a resource to you as primary care providers and increase your common tool set in being able to manage common ENT issues and concerns.

I also have many words of thanks to extend. It has been an honor and a joy to serve as the guest editor for this issue of *Primary Care: Clinics in Office Practice*, and I am immensely grateful to Elsevier and to Dr Heidelbaugh, Nitesh Barthwal, and the editorial staff at Elsevier for this opportunity. It has been a pure joy. I also want to thank each one of our contributing authors, who have worked tirelessly and have provided us with information that is both clinically relevant and scholarly. I also want to thank the Department of Family Medicine at Rutgers Robert Wood Johnson University

Prim Care Clin Office Pract 52 (2025) xv–xvi
https://doi.org/10.1016/j.pop.2024.12.001
0095-4543/25/© 2024 Published by Elsevier Inc.

primarycare.theclinics.com

Hospital Somerset and the leadership at Rutgers Robert Wood Johnson Somerset Family Practice, whose support was critical in this project. I am immensely grateful.

DISCLOSURES

The author does not have any disclosures of any commercial or financial conflicts nor any funding sources.

Donna M. Kaminski, DO, MPH, FAAFP
Department of Family Medicine
Rutgers Robert Wood Johnson
University Hospital Somerset
Somerset Family Practice
Family Medicine Residency Program
128 Rehill Avenue
Somerville, NJ 08876, USA

E-mail address:
donna.kaminski@rwjbh.org

REFERENCES

1. Patel EA, Poulson TA, Shah M, et al. Evaluation of wait times for otolaryngology appointments in Illinois. OTO Open 2023;7(3):e63.
2. Sorichetti BD, Pauwels J, Jacobs TB, et al. High frequency of otolaryngology/ENT encounters in Canadian primary care despite low medical undergraduate experiences. Can Med Educ J 2022;13(1):86–9.

Otitides
Acute and Chronic Otitis Media and Externa

Jennifer Bustamante, DO[a,b,*], Tony Tran, DO[c],
Carlos R. Rodriguez, MD[a,b]

KEYWORDS

- Otoscopy • Earache • Otalgia • Tympanostomy tube • Otitis media • Otitis externa
- Antibiotics

KEY POINTS

- Acute otitis media (AOM) is more common in children than adults and leads to frequent antibiotic use.
- AOM-related pain (otalgia) can prompt parents to seek treatment for their children.
- Overdiagnosis of AOM leads to unnecessary antibiotic use, contributing to antibiotic resistance.
- Differentiating between AOM and otitis media with effusion is imperative to determine whether watchful waiting versus antibiotic treatment is indicated.
- Acute otitis externa is an inflammatory ear canal condition commonly caused by bacterial infection, mainly *Pseudomonas aeruginosa* and *Staphylococcus aureus*.

INTRODUCTION

Otitis media (OM) and otitis externa (OE) are distinct yet common ear conditions affecting a significant portion of the population across all age groups. The clinical presentation of these conditions is diverse, ranging from subtle or absent symptoms in cases of otitis media with effusion (OME) to acute pain and discomfort associated with acute otitis media (AOM), chronic suppurative otitis media (CSOM), and OE.

Despite their prevalence, OM and OE pathophysiology involves a complex interplay of microbial invasion, host immune response, and environmental factors. The complexity of treating otitides highlights the importance of a comprehensive approach to prevention, proper diagnosis, and treatment. The authors aim to explore the current

[a] NSUKPCOM Family Medicine Residency Program, Evara Health; [b] Department of Family Medicine, Evara Health, 14100 58 Street N, Clearwater, FL 33760, USA; [c] PGY1, Department of Family Medicine, Evara Health, Clearwater, FL, USA
* Corresponding author. Department of Family Medicine, Evara Health, 14100 58 Street N, Clearwater, FL 33760.
E-mail address: jebustamante@hcnetwork.org

Prim Care Clin Office Pract 52 (2025) 1–14
https://doi.org/10.1016/j.pop.2024.09.003   **primarycare.theclinics.com**
0095-4543/25/© 2024 Elsevier Inc. All rights reserved, including those for text and data mining, AI training, and similar technologies.

OM and OE guidelines, highlighting the latest advances in treatment methods and the ongoing challenges in managing these ubiquitous ear conditions.

ANATOMY OF THE EAR

The ear is a sensory organ responsible for hearing and maintaining balance. It consists of 3 parts: the internal ear, the middle ear, and the external ear. The middle ear is an air-filled space composed of the tympanic membrane (TM) that posteriorly houses 3 auditory ossicles (malleus, incus, and stapes). The bones amplify and transmit high-amplitude, low-force sound waves into low-amplitude, high-force vibrations from the TM to the oval window. Beyond the oval window, the middle ear is also connected to the nasopharynx by the Eustachian tube, allowing fluid drainage and pressure equalization from the middle ear to the outer environment.[1]

Acute Otitis Media

AOM is defined as the sudden onset of inflammation or infection of the middle ear resulting in the accumulation of purulent or suppurative fluid behind the tympanic membrane. OM is among the most common pediatric diagnoses in primary care, ranking among the leading diagnoses contributing to antibiotic overuse and antibiotic resistance.[2] In the United States, over 5 million cases of AOM and 2.2 million cases of OME are reported annually.[3] Although AOM may occur at any age, most cases occur in young children aged 6 to 24 months.[4] The incidence peaks at 1 year of age and declines after the age of 5.[5]

ETIOLOGY AND RISK FACTORS

AOM is caused by fluid accumulation in the middle ear, leading to rapid inflammation and dysfunction in the Eustachian tube (ET) anatomy, in decreased fluid drainage, and increased inner ear pressure. Inflammation of the ET is often triggered by a viral or bacterial pathogen or allergens, resulting in fluid retention and purulent effusion in the middle ear. A shortened ET in children increases the risk of otitis infections.[6]

Various risk factors can influence otitis media. Understanding these factors is essential for prevention and early management. **Box 1** summarizes several contributing risk factors suspected of increasing the predisposition of AOM.

Viral upper respiratory tract infections (URIs) pose a significant risk for AOM. URIs caused by respiratory syncytial virus, influenza virus, picornavirus, coronavirus, human metapneumovirus, and adenovirus are the most common viral causes of AOM.[7] During a viral infection, bacteria migrate from the nasopharynx to the middle ear, causing AOM.[8] Bacterial pathogens, such as Streptococcus pneumoniae and Haemophilus influenzae, are believed to be the primary agents. Streptococcus pneumoniae is responsible for half of all cases of AOM, and the presence of penicillin-resistant strains lead to treatment failure and increased recurrence of AOM.[9] Non-typeable Haemophilus influenzae, Moraxella catarrhalis, and Staphylococcus aureus also have notable roles in the pathogenesis of AOM.[10] Conjugate vaccines effective against pneumococcus and Haemophilis influenzae could potentially reduce the burden of AOM in early infancy; however, their impact on all-cause AOM remains uncertain, based on evidence of low to moderate certainty. Moreover, there is no evidence of a beneficial effect on all-cause AOM in high-risk infants beyond early infancy or in older children with a history of respiratory illness.[11–13]

Genetic factors are not just a side note in the pathogenesis of acute otitis media (AOM); they also play a significant role in influencing both the susceptibility to infection

Box 1
Risk factors for acute otitis media
Male Gender
Age under 5 years old
Premature birth (less than 37 weeks gestation)
Immunodeficiency–congenital, human immunodeficiency virus
Diabetes
Anatomic abnormalities of the palate and associated musculature
Down syndrome
Gastroesophageal reflux
Allergies
Family members with a history or recurrence of acute otitis media Indigenous populations such as Native Americans, the Alaskan, Canadian, and Greenland Inuit and Australian Aborigines
Large daycare attendance
Parental smoking exposure
Recurrent Upper Respiratory Infections
Presence of cochlear implant
Seasonality–Winter and Early Spring
Pacifier use
Supine bottle feeding
Lack of breast-feeding during infancy
Information from references:[5,16,24,40,44–46]

and the severity of the condition. Research has identified several genetic variants and polymorphisms associated with an increased risk of AOM, including variations in tumor necrosis factor-α and interleukin-6 and interleukin-10 alleles altering cytokine production, exacerbating inflammation, and increasing the frequency of AOM episodes.[14–16] This underscores the importance of genetic research in understanding and potentially preventing AOM.

CLINICAL PRESENTATION AND DIAGNOSIS

AOM primarily affects infants and children, who may initially exhibit otalgia, followed by irritability, poor appetite, sleep disturbances, and ear tugging due to severe pain. **Box 2** summarizes the most common presenting symptoms of AOM.

The American Academy of Pediatrics (AAP) offers evidence-based clinical practice guidelines focusing on diagnosing and managing AOM in children. Key points covered in **Table 1** include strategies for managing ear pain, guidance on when to observe versus prescribe antibiotics, recommendations for appropriate antibiotic choices, preventive measures, and addressing recurrent AOM. These guidelines aim to assist primary care clinicians by providing a structured framework for clinical decision-making, emphasizing that they serve as a valuable resource but do not replace individual clinical judgment. Accurate diagnosis is crucial for the proper management of AOM and

Box 2
Common symptoms of acute otitis media
Otalgia
Ear rubbing or tugging
Night restlessness
Fussiness or irritability
Decreased hearing
Fever
Otorrhea
Headache
Vomiting
Diarrhea
Loss of appetite
Less active or playful
Information from references:[26,47,48]

OME. AOM diagnosis requires a thorough history, clinical assessment, and evidence of middle ear effusion.[17]

The diagnosis of AOM and OME should start with an otoscopic inspection of the TM. This is shown in **Fig. 1**A, B[18] Medical professionals should note any abnormal TM characteristics as described in **Table 2**. This should be followed by a pneumatic otoscopy to assess for middle ear effusion. No laboratory testing or imaging is required for a diagnosis unless it is to confirm or exclude a congenital or systemic disease. The diagnostic criteria for AOM include moderate to severe bulging of the tympanic membrane, new onset of otorrhea, or mild bulging associated with recent ear pain or erythema.[19]

Each examination should meticulously describe the TM, dividing it into 4 quadrants upon visualization. This comprehensive approach considers the following 4 TM characteristics: Color, Position, Mobility, and Perforation; a normal TM, as shown in **Fig. 1**C, is neutral, not bulging or retracted, and pearly gray, translucent, and unperforated. This detailed description of the TM is a crucial part of every examination, providing a comprehensive understanding of the ear condition.[20]

The absence of tympanic membrane movement during pneumatic otoscopy is the primary diagnostic tool for detecting AOM and OME, highlighting the importance of thorough cerumen removal from the external auditory canal. This method boasts a sensitivity and specificity of 70% to 90% compared to myringotomy.[21] However, it is crucial to perform the procedure correctly, as many medical professionals may not do so, potentially resulting in misdiagnosis.

The American Academy of Otolaryngology-Head and Neck Surgery (AAO-HNS) updated guidelines on OME and recommended tympanometry screening for children aged 4 to 6 years at the start of school and 1 year later. Tympanometry failure, indicated by middle ear pressure above −200 daPa or a flat tympanometric curve, requires further assessment, especially if accompanied by a 20-dB hearing loss at specific frequencies. Retesting after 2 months is advised for unilateral or bilateral tympanometry failure, with persistent failure warranting immediate physician evaluation, including hearing, speech, and language assessment and appropriate therapy.[22]

Table 1
2013 American academy of pediatrics otitis media guidelines

	Current Recommendations
Diagnostic Criteria	It necessitates significant bulging of the tympanic membrane, the emergence of otorrhea unrelated to external ear inflammation, or slight bulging of the eardrum coupled with a recent onset of ear pain (within 48 hours) or erythema. There should be objective evidence of middle ear effusion.
Initial Management of acute otitis media (AOM)	Should include adequate analgesia for all children and adults with acetaminophen or non-steroidal anti-inflammatory drugs
Non-Severe AOM (Bilateral) in 6–23-month-old (Unilateral) in 6–23-month-old Age 2 y or older	Mild otalgia for <48 hours Temperature: 39°C Should be started on a 10-d course of high dose of antibiotics Consider watchful waiting with close follow-up or a 10-day course of antibiotic therapy after a decision-making discussion with parents Watchful waiting with close follow-up and treatment with analgesics along with providing a safety net antibiotic prescription if symptoms persist if unable to follow up and symptoms persist within 48–72 hours Or Oral analgesia and High-dose amoxicillin for 5–7 days
Antibiotics for severe AOM Unilateral or Bilateral	Children aged at least 6 months with severe signs or symptoms (moderate or severe otalgia; otalgia for 48 h or longer; temperature 39°C or higher):Should be started on a 10-d course of antibiotics.
Choice of antibiotic	High-dose amoxicillin (80–90 mg per kg per day in 2 divided doses) is preferred as a first choice unless the child received it within 30 days, has concurrent purulent conjunctivitis, or is allergic to penicillin.
Second-line antibiotics	If the amoxicillin criteria are unmet, prescribe an antibiotic with additional beta-lactamase coverage, such as amoxicillin-clavulanate.
Re-evaluation in patient with unresolved symptoms	If symptoms worsen or do not respond to initial antibiotic treatment within 48–72 hours, change treatment if otitis media is present. Consider intramuscular ceftriaxone (Rocephin), clindamycin, or tympanocentesis if symptoms worsen despite adequate therapy.
Management of recurrent AOM ≥ 3 episodes in 6 mo or 4 in 1 year with ≥ 1 episode in the proceeding 6 months	Tympanostomy tubes (TTs) reduce the frequency of AOM episodes, decrease the risk of infections, and prevent persistent middle ear effusion (MEE); prophylactic antibiotics are not recommended; referral to otolaryngologist may be necessary

(continued on next page)

Table 1 (continued)	
	Current Recommendations
Persistent MEE	Monitor for 3–6 month intervals with hearing tests for effusions lasting longer than 3 months or any signs of speech or developmental delay.
Vaccination recommendations	Updated pneumococcal conjugate vaccine and annual influenza vaccine recommended for all children
Promotion of breastfeeding	Encourage exclusive breastfeeding for 6 months or longer

Information from references:[7,10,17]

Alternative diagnostic methods like acoustic reflectometry have limited acceptance among otolaryngologists due to challenges in establishing interpretation standards. Instead, audiometry is a suitable method to assess middle ear effusions. Tympanocentesis is the preferred technique for identifying middle ear effusion and confirming bacterial infection, but it is underused in primary care settings. It enhances diagnostic accuracy and guides treatment, potentially reducing unnecessary interventions in recurrent cases.[10,23] Detecting OME is crucial, as it is often associated with allergies, upper respiratory tract infection, or Eustachian tube dysfunction. Observing OME for 3 months is recommended, as antibiotics are not proven to treat middle ear effusions.

CURRENT TREATMENT OPTIONS

The initial approach to treating acute otitis media begins with properly addressing symptomatology, most notably otalgia, with topical or oral analgesics (acetaminophen or non-steroidal anti-inflammatory drugs [NSAIDs]) for mild to moderate ear pain, while severe pain may require narcotics. The AAP treatment guidelines are noted in **Table 3**. Observation and pain management for 2 to 3 days without antibiotics is recommended for children aged 6 to 23 months with unilateral acute otitis media.. Antibiotics should be reserved for severe cases or children under 2 years old with bilateral acute otitis media, regardless of symptoms.[17] A watch-and-wait approach may be acceptable for 2 out of 3 children, with a subsequent follow-up visit for those whose symptoms

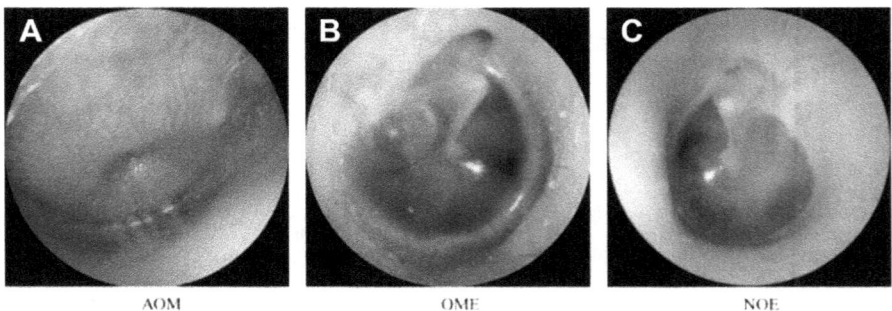

AOM   OME   NOE

Fig. 1. Otoscopy images of the tympanic membrane with acute otitis media (A), otitis media with effusion (B), and no effusion (C). (Source[18] Sundgaard JV, Harte J, Bray P, Laugesen S, Kamide Y, Tanaka C, Paulsen RR, Christensen AN.Med Image Anal. 2021 Jul;71:102034. https://creativecommons.org/licenses/by/4.0.)

Table 2
Classic characteristics of tympanic membrane in otitis media with effusion (OME), acute otitis media (AOM), eustachian tube dysfunction (ETD)

Color	OME—opaque, yellow or blue tympanic membrane (TM) AOM—dark pink or light red Crying fever, cough or blowing nose–Hyperemia
Position	OME—Retracted or in the neutral position AOM—Bulging
Mobility	ETD—TM movement with negative pressure OME—Slight movement of TM with positive and negative pressure AOM—No movement of TM
Perforation	Single to multiple perforations

Information from reference:[20]

does not improve after 48 to 72 hours. An alternative is to provide a safety net antibiotic prescription for those unable to follow up or whose symptoms worsen.[24]

Amoxicillin 80 to 90 mg/kg/day divided every 12 hours for a total of 10 days is the first-line treatment for AOM, effective in both children and adults is amoxicillin-clavulanate (80–90 mg/kg/day-6.4 mg/kg/day) divided every 12 hours recommended for recurrent cases, infections concurrent with conjunctivitis, or recent amoxicillin use within 30 days.[19] For patients allergic to penicillin, alternative empiric antibiotics may include as follows:

- Clarithromycin (15 mg/kg per day in 2 divided doses) or azithromycin (10 mg/kg single dose)
- Cefuroxine axetil (30 mg/kg/day in 2 divided doses)
- Cefdinir (14 mg/kg/day in 1 or 2 divided doses)
- Cefpodoxime (10 mg/kg/day in 2 divided doses)
- Intramuscular (IM) ceftriaxone (a single IM injection of 50 mg/kg for 3 consecutive days).

No oral/intramuscular cephalosporin is superior to amoxicillin.[25,26]

Those patients with 4 or more episodes of AOM in the past 12 months should undergo a myringotomy with tube placement or tympanocentesis with fluid aspiration for both diagnostic and therapeutic effects by reducing middle ear pain and pressure. However, they do not shorten effusion duration or AOM recurrence.[27] Recurrent AOM

Table 3
Topical Agents used in the treatment of acute otitis externa

Medication	Dosing	Non-Ototoxic
Acetic acid 2% (VoSol)	4 to 6 times daily	No
Acetic acid 2%, hydrocortisone 1% (VoSol HC)	4 to 6 times daily	No
Neomycin, polymyxin B, hydrocortisone (Costisporin)	3 to 4 times daily	No
Ciprofloxacin 0.2%, hydrocortisone 1% (Cipro HC)	Twice daily	No
Ciprofloxacin 0.3%, dexamethasone 0.1% (Ciprodex)	Twice daily	Yes
Ofloxacin 0.3%	Once daily	Yes
Ciprofloxacin 0.2%	Twice daily	Yes

Information from references:[34,49,50]

may necessitate tympanostomy tube insertion for pressure equalization and assist with middle ear drainage by reducing the risk of future infections.[28,29] Tympanostomy tubes are safe but may be complicated by ear tube retraction or displacement.[30] A 2023 Cochrane review on antibiotic use for AOM concluded, based on a meta-analysis of several studies, that antibiotics did not significantly reduce the number of children with pain at 24 hours or decrease the occurrence of late AOM recurrences compared to placebo. However, antibiotics slightly lowered the incidence of eardrum perforations and AOM in the initially unaffected ear. Despite reducing abnormal tympanometry findings in the short term, antibiotics had limited long-term benefits. While data on rare complications like mastoiditis were lacking, antibiotics led to adverse effects such as diarrhea, vomiting, and rash, making it challenging to balance their modest benefits against potential harms, particularly in mild cases of AOM in high-income countries.[31]

COMPLICATIONS AND THEIR MANAGEMENT

Recurrent acute otitis media or persistent middle ear effusions can progress to chronic serous otitis media (CSOM), causing lasting inflammation with otorrhea. CSOM often leads to mild to moderate hearing loss, affecting around 61% of patients. Recent studies support oral and topical ciprofloxacin for CSOM treatment, underlining the need for a culture to guide therapy and prevent severe complications like facial paralysis, brain abscesses, and permanent hearing loss.[32] Mastoiditis, a complication of CSOM, requires prompt clinical examination, computed tomography (CT) or MRI, and treatment with intravenous antibiotics or surgical debridement to prevent severe complications like facial paralysis, meningitis, or sepsis. A cholesteatoma, a benign skin growth in the middle ear and mastoid process, can also develop resulting in malodorous ear discharge, increased inner ear pressure, dizziness, and hearing impairment, often necessitating surgical intervention.[33]

Otitis Externa

OE is a common inflammatory condition affecting the ear canal, also known as "swimmer's ear." It is often caused by an infectious agent due to increased water exposure in tropical climates or during summer months. OE can be acute (less than 6 weeks) or chronic (more than 3 months).[34]

EPIDEMIOLOGY AND RISK FACTORS

Acute otitis externa (AOE) is an ear canal inflammation that causes more than 500,000 health care visits annually in the United States.[35] It's the most common waterborne disease. It is more common during the summer, affecting mostly 7- to 12-year-olds and people living in humid tropical areas.[36] There's no gender predominance, and 10% of individuals will experience this condition at some point in their lifetime.[34]

Several risk factors increase the risk of AOE. These risk factors include anatomic abnormalities (stenosis of the canal, hairy canals, and exostoses), dermatologic conditions (eczema, psoriasis, and seborrhea), obstruction (inclusion cysts, cerumen impaction, and foreign bodies), changes in the integrity of cerumen or epithelium (excessive cerumen removal, instrumentation or scratching of the canal, and the use of earplugs, earbuds or hearing aids), water exposure, and miscellaneous causes such as soap irritation, purulent otorrhea as a sequela from otitis media, and having type A blood.[35] Of all these, the most common risk factor is swimming and exposure to any form of water, including sweating or humidity.[37]

PATHOPHYSIOLOGY

Cerumen-producing glands and hair follicles surround the external auditory canal. Otitis externa is an inflammatory process due to pH changes and disruption of protective factors in the auditory canal. The pH in the canal usually ranges from 5 to 5.7 and inhibits bacterial growth due to its hydrophobic properties.[38] Cerumen is one of these protective factors and promotes an acidic environment that inhibits bacterial and fungal growth. However, moisture build-up from epithelial damage and wax loss can alter the pH levels, leading to bacterial overgrowth.[34] *Pseudomonas aeruginosa* and *Staphlococcus aureus* are the most prevalent, accounting for 90% of cases.[37]

CLINICAL PRESENTATION

A hallmark of AOE is ear pain that can be reproduced with movement of the tragus. The most common presenting symptoms are pain, itching, and a feeling of fullness in the ear, which can be worsened by manipulating the temporomandibular joint, tragus, or pinna.[36] Patients may often complain that the pain worsens at night.[33] The pain can be accompanied by otorrhea, erythema, itching, swelling of the canal, and hearing changes.[38] The symptoms usually appear within 48 hours of disease onset.

DIAGNOSIS

Diagnosing AOE relies on an accurate physical examination and medical history. The ear canal and the tympanic membrane should be inspected using an otoscope or otomicroscope during the physical examination.[39] The AAO-HNS proposed specific criteria for diagnosing this condition. These criteria include the following symptoms and presentation: sudden onset of symptoms, usually within 48 hours in the past 3 weeks, signs of ear canal inflammation such as tenderness on the movement of the pinna or tragus, diffuse canal edema or erythema, ear pain, itching, a feeling of fullness in the ear, and, in some cases, jaw pain or hearing loss. The diagnosis may also include otorrhea, rupture of the tympanic membrane, cellulitis, or lymphadenitis involvement.[35]

TREATMENT

Uncomplicated AOE treatment encompasses ear canal cleansing, topical antiseptic, antibiotics, and analgesia.[38] Structural defects in the tympanic membrane should be ruled out before rinsing with water or saline. Avoid using cotton swabs to prevent bacterial invasion. Ear canal cleaning involves the removal of cerumen and exudate, which may contain toxins that aid in maintaining the inflammatory process. The cleaning process involves microscopic visualization and suction or the use of an aural hook by an experienced clinician to avoid injury. The cleaning process helps topical drugs work better by removing toxins like Pseudomonas exotoxin A.

Topical antiseptics can effectively remove moisture, decrease edema, and reduce acid production, thereby inhibiting the growth of bacteria attributed to the alcohol content in the preparations. Various antiseptics are on the market, including aluminum acetate, silver nitrate, N-cholorotaurine, fuchsin, eosin, and acetic acid. After 7 days of treatment, acetic acid showed comparable effectiveness to antibiotic or corticosteroid drops. However, after 2 to 3 weeks of use, it was significantly less effective.[38]

Topical antimicrobials are the mainstay of treatment for this condition. A meta-analysis of randomized control trials and a systematic review of 26 combinations of topical agents showed no significant difference in outcome, with most patients experiencing clinical resolution within 7 to 10 days regardless of which agent or combination was used.[40] If there is a perforation in the tympanic membrane, topical medications with aminoglycosides or isopropyl alcohol should be avoided due to ototoxicity. Non-sterile ear preparations should also be avoided in the presence of a TM perforation. Quinolones are the only Food and Drug Association-approved topical agent for treating OE with a TM perforation.[41]

Topical therapy is more effective than oral antibiotics as it delivers higher concentrations of antimicrobials, reducing bacterial resistance risk. In most cases of AOE, oral antibiotics should not be used. However, despite this, 20% to 40% of patients are still prescribed oral antibiotics in addition to topical therapy. Oral antibiotics are ineffective against the most common pathogens, including *Pseudomonas aeruginosa* and *Staphylococcus aureus*. Oral antibiotics can be used for patients with uncontrolled diabetes or those who are immunocompromised and unable to apply topical agents. Oral antibiotics are indicated when the infection spreads beyond the ear canal. In such cases, a referral to an otolaryngologist may be needed.[35,41]

Notably, a 2023 systematic review involving 3 meta-analyses demonstrated no significant difference in measured outcomes for antibiotics compared to non-antibiotic treatments like antiseptics and steroids. This study was consistent with prior meta-analyses that found topical antiseptics were not inferior to antibiotics when managing AOE. This provides an opportunity to contribute to antimicrobial stewardship by reducing antibiotic use and, thus, resistance.[42]

The assessment and treatment of pain is also a key factor in managing AOE. The AAO-HNS established guidelines in 2014 that were affirmed by the American Academy of Family Physicians in 2019. The adequate management of pain has been shown to help patients return to normal activities sooner and increase comfort. Analgesic options include acetaminophen and NSAIDs with fixed intervals rather than as-needed dosing. Topical analgesics have been withdrawn from the market, particularly otic benzocaine in 2015, due to the dilution potential of antibiotic drops and unknown ototoxicity associated with use.[35]

MONITORING

Patients should experience an improvement in symptoms within 2 to 3 days of beginning treatment. However, if symptoms do not improve, an ear culture may be obtained to help discern between bacterial and fungal etiologies and help tailor treatment further. Other possibilities, such as cellulitis or contact dermatitis, should be considered if symptoms persist despite adequate treatment. Based on epidemiologic data, only 3% of patients require a second evaluation by an otolaryngologist.[26] Following up within 2 weeks of beginning treatment is appropriate to assess progress and resolution. If there is a concern for malignant otitis externa, a referral to an otolaryngologist is necessary. Other considerations for referral include the primary provider not being comfortable managing a severely edematous canal with lavage, placing a wick, or additional removal of debris.[35]

COMPLICATIONS

Malignant otitis externa (MOE) is a rare but serious complication caused by an infection of the auditory canal and surrounding structures, including the bone. *Pseudomonas aeruginosa* is usually associated with 90% of the cases and is most seen in elderly diabetics or those with human immunodeficiency virus. MOE consists of severe ear pain, high fever, granulation tissue along the external auditory canal, vertigo, meningeal signs, and cranial nerve palsies. A CT scan can confirm the diagnosis and determine the extent of the disease. MRI can identify soft-tissue abnormalities and retrocondylar fat infiltration. Treatment usually involves surgical debridement and parenteral antibiotics. The first-line therapy is ciprofloxacin, 750 mg twice daily orally, for at least 4 weeks.[26]

PREVENTION

Limiting water exposure, retention of moisture, acutely recurrent cerumen impaction, minimizing trauma using cotton swabs and hearing aids, and preventing the introduction of any foreign body will certainly limit the recurrence of cases.[36] In cases where patients intend to spend significant time around water, the ear canal should be kept dry and would benefit from using a drying mechanism, such as a hair dryer, to keep the canal free of moisture. Head-tilt maneuvers can also help dry out the ear canal.[38] To completely prevent canal moisture, a well-fitted earplug can be used. Despite no trial reflecting effectiveness, some recommend the use of acetic acid 2% solution as a preventive measure.[35]

Chronic Otitis Externa

Chronic otitis externa is a persistent ear canal inflammation that lasts more than 3 months or occurs more than 4 times a year. It can cause itching and hearing loss. There is rarely any pain involved. Chronic inflammation can lead to fibrosis of the ear canal, which can cause either redness due to moisture in the eczematous form or a dry, scaly, and shiny canal in the seborrheic form; this can lead to acute inflammation when patients manipulate their ear canal.[38] As sequelae of chronic inflammation, a fibrous scar can begin to form at the medial border of the ear canal, and associated fibrotic changes can result in conductive hearing loss from obstruction because of fibrotic plug formation.[39] If the ear canal is stenotic, a canaloplasty can be performed to widen it.[38]

Chronic inflammation can cause extracranial and intracranial complications. Extracranial complications may include vestibular/balance problems, eardrum perforation with otorrhea, hearing impairment, cholesteatoma, tympanosclerosis, and mastoiditis. Intracranial complications may cause serious health issues such as sinus thrombosis, subdural empyema, and abscess with involvement to the epidural or brain. Mastoiditis can lead to bone involvement with either osteitis or periostitis. If diagnosed, treatment may involve intravenous antibiotics and surgery following diagnosis confirmation with CT or MRI.[26]

There are no clear or explicit recommendations for treating chronic otitis externa, and available randomized control trials on drug therapy are lacking. What is effective is keeping the ear canal dry and free of potential irritants like soap to help promote the canal's original balanced state and a conducive environment for cerumen production. To reduce inflammation, you can use topical treatments. You can also try using alcohol or a corticosteroid solution to help reduce swelling in the ear canal. It is important to get a culture to identify any pathogens. If the culture is positive, you will need antibiotics or antifungal medication. If treatment is resistant, oral corticosteroids can be an effective alternative and tacrolimus has been documented to be beneficial.[39]

COMPLEMENTARY TREATMENT FOR OTITIDES

Osteopathic Manipulative Treatment (OMT) can effectively address otitis media and otitis externa by using gentle techniques to correct biomechanical restrictions and improve Eustachian tube function. Techniques such as the Galbreath Maneuver and the Auricular Drainage Technique facilitate fluid and lymphatic drainage from the middle ear. A study in the *Archives of Pediatrics and Adolescent Medicine* found that OMT, when used alongside routine care, resulted in fewer episodes of acute otitis media (AOM), fewer surgical procedures, and increased normal tympanograms without adverse reactions.[43] While these results are promising, further research is necessary to confirm OMT's efficacy.

CLINICS CARE POINTS

- Both AOM and OE necessitate comprehensive approaches to prevention, diagnosis, and treatment.
- It is important to focus on symptom relief and cautious antibiotic use when treating AOM.
- OE management involves ear canal cleansing, topical antimicrobials, and avoiding unnecessary oral antibiotics.

DISCLOSURE

The authors have nothing to disclose.

REFERENCES

1. Moore KL, Dalley AF, AAM R. Clinically oriented anatomy. Philadelphia etc: Wolters Kluwer; 2018. p. 966–73.
2. Célind J, Södermark L, Hjalmarson O. Adherence to treatment guidelines for acute otitis media in children. The necessity of an effective strategy of guideline implementation. Int J Pediatr Otorhinolaryngol 2014;78:1128–32.
3. Suaya JA, Gessner BD, Fung S, et al. Acute otitis media, antimicrobial prescriptions, and medical expenses among children in the United States during 2011–2016. Vaccine 2018;36:7479–86.
4. Rettig EM, Tunkel DE. Acute otitis media in children. *Infections of the ears, nose, throat, and sinuses.* Cham, Switzerland: Springer International Publishing AG; 2018. p. 45–55.
5. Baraibar R. Incidence and risk factors of acute otitis media in children. Clin Microbiol Infection 1997;3(Suppl 3):S13–22.
6. Tong S, Amand C, Kieffer A, et al. Trends in healthcare utilization and costs associated with acute otitis media in the United States during 2008–2014. BMC Health Serv Res 2018;18:1–10.
7. Lobb B, Lee MC, McElheny CL, et al. Genomic classification and antimicrobial resistance profiling of *Streptococcus pneumoniae* and *Haemophilus influenzae* isolates associated with pediatric otitis media and upper respiratory infection. BMC Infect Dis 2023;23:596.
8. Arrieta A, Singh J. Management of recurrent and persistent acute otitis media: new options with familiar antibiotics. Pediatr Infect Dis J 2004;23(2):S115–24.
9. Massa HM, Cripps AW, Lehmann D. Otitis media: viruses, bacteria, biofilms, and vaccines. Med J Aust 2009;191(9):S44–9.
10. Ngo CC, Massa HM, McMonagle BA, et al. Predominant bacterial and viral otopathogens identified within the respiratory tract and middle ear of urban Australian children experiencing otitis media are diversely distributed. Front Cell Infect Microbiol 2022;12:14.
11. Straetemans MM, Sanders EAM, Veenhoven RH, et al. Pneumococcal vaccines for preventing otitis media. Cochrane Database Syst Rev 2004;1:CD001480.

12. Fireman B, Black SB, Shinefield Henry R, et al. Impact of the pneumococcal conjugate vaccine on otitis media. Pediatr Infect Dis J 2003;22(1):10–6.
13. Intakorn P, Sonsuwan N, Noknu S, et al. *Haemophilus influenzae* type b as an important cause of culture-positive acute otitis media in young children in Thailand: a tympanocentesis-based, multi-center, cross-sectional study. BMC Pediatr 2014;14:157.
14. Jamal A, Alsabea A, Tarakmeh M, et al. Etiology, diagnosis, complications, and management of acute otitis media in children. Cureus 2022;14(8):e28019.
15. Emonts M, Veenhoven RH, Wiertsema SP, et al. Genetic polymorphisms in immunoresponse genes *TNFA, IL6, IL10,* and *TLR4* are associated with recurrent acute otitis media. Pediatrics 2007;120(4):814–23.
16. Geng R, Wang Q, Chen E, et al. Current understanding of host genetics of otitis media. Front Genet 2020;10:1395.
17. Bradley M, Bacharouch A, Hart-Johnson T, et al. Adopting otitis media practice guidelines increases adherence within a large primary care network. J Paediatr Child Health 2021;57(7):1054–9.
18. Sundgaard JV, Harte J, Bray P, et al. Med Image Anal 2021;71:102034.
19. Shaikh N, Hoberman A, Kaleida PH, et al. Otoscopic signs of otitis media. Pediatr Infect Dis J 2011;30(10):822–6.
20. Watters GW, Jones JE, Freeland AP. The predictive value of tympanometry in the diagnosis of middle ear effusion. Clin Otolayngol Allied Sci 1997;22(4):343–5.
21. Rosenfeld RM, Shin JJ, Schwartz SR, et al. Clinical practice guideline: otitis media with effusion (update). Otolaryngology-Head Neck Surg (Tokyo) 2016;154:S1–41.
22. Lambert M. AAO-HNS releases updated guideline on management of otitis media with effusion. Am Fam Physician 2016;94(9):747–9.
23. Harmes KM, Blackwood RA, Burrows HL, et al. Otitis media: diagnosis and treatment. Am Fam Physician 2013;88(7):435–40. Erratum in: Am Fam Physician. 2014 Mar 1;89(5):318. Dosage error in article text.
24. Brinker DL, MacGeorge EL, Hackman N. Diagnostic accuracy, prescription behavior, and watchful waiting efficacy for pediatric acute otitis media. Clin Pediatr (Phila) 2019;58(1):60–5.
25. Lieberthal AS, Carroll AE, Chonmaitree T, et al. The diagnosis and management of acute otitis media. Pediatrics 2013;131(3):e964–99.
26. Lee H, Kim J, Nguyen V. Ear infections: otitis externa and otitis media. Prim Care 2013;40(3):671–86.
27. Gonzalez C, Arnold JE, Woody EA, et al. Prevention of recurrent acute otitis media: chemoprophylaxis versus tympanostomy tubes. Laryngoscope 1986;96:1330–4.
28. Lous J, Ryborg CT, Thomsen JL. A systematic review of the effect of tympanostomy tubes in children with recurrent acute otitis media. Int J Pediatr Otorhinolaryngol 2011;75:1058–61.
29. Lau L, Mick P, Nunez DA. Grommets (ventilation tubes) for recurrent acute otitis media in children [WITHDRAWN]. Cochrane Database Syst Rev 2018;4:0.
30. Rosenfeld RM, Bhaya MH, Bower CM, et al. Impact of tympanostomy tubes on child quality of life. Arch Otolaryngol Head Neck Surg 2000;126:585–92.
31. Venekamp RP, Sanders SL, Glasziou PP, et al. Antibiotics for acute otitis media in children. Cochrane Database Syst Rev 2023;11(11):CD000219.
32. Renukananda GS. A comparative study of oral and topical ciprofloxacin in the treatment of tubotympanic chronic suppurative otitis media. Pakistan Journal of Medical and Health Sciences 2020;14(1):315–8.

33. Acute otitis externa (Swimmer's Ear). Am Fam Physician 2023;107(2).
34. Medina-Blasini Y, Sharman T. Otitis Externa. In: StatPearls. Treasure island (FL): StatPearls Publishing; 2023.
35. Jackson EA, Geer K. Acute Otitis Externa: Rapid Evidence Review. Am Fam Physician 2023;107(2):145–51.
36. Plum AW, Wong M. An Overview of Acute Otitis Externa. Otolaryngol Clin North Am 2023;56(5):891–6.
37. Nieratschker M, Haas M, Lucic M, et al. The association between acute otitis externa-related emergency department visits and extreme weather events in a temperate continental climate. Int J Hyg Environ Health 2024;255:114274.
38. Wiegand S, Berner R, Schneider A, et al. Otitis Externa. Dtsch Arztebl Int 2019; 116(13):224–34.
39. Wipperman J. Otitis externa. Prim Care 2014;41(1):1–9.
40. Schaefer P, Baugh RF. Acute otitis externa: an update. Am Fam Physician 2012; 86(11):1055–61.
41. Mughal Z, Swaminathan R, Al-Deerawi HB, et al, March 27. A Systematic Review of Antibiotic Prescription for Acute Otitis Externa. Cureus 2021;13(3):e14149.
42. Di Traglia R, Tudor-Green B, Muzaffar J, et al. Antibiotics versus nonantibiotic treatments for acute otitis externa: A systematic review and meta-analysis. Clin Otolaryngol 2023;48(6):841–62.
43. Mills MV, Henley CE, Barnes LLB, et al. The Use of Osteopathic Manipulative Treatment as Adjuvant Therapy in Children With Recurrent Acute Otitis Media. Arch Pediatr Adolesc Med 2003;157(9):861–6.
44. Dickson G. Acute otitis media. Prim Care 2014;41(1):11–8.
45. Gaddey HL, Wright MT, Nelson TN. Otitis Media: Rapid Evidence Review. Am Fam Physician 2019;100(6):350–6.
46. Szmuilowicz J, Young R. Infections of the Ear. Emerg Med Clin North Am 2019; 37(1):1–9.
47. Danishyar A, Ashurst JV. Acute Otitis Media. In: StatPearls. Treasure Island (FL): StatPearls Publishing; 2023.
48. Qureishi A, Lee Y, Belfield K. etal. Update on otitis media- prevention and treatment. Infect Drug Resist 2014;7:15–24.
49. Rosenfeld RM, Schwartz SR, Cannon CR, et al. Clinical practice guideline: acute otitis externa [published correction appears in Otolaryngol Head Neck Surg. 2014;150(3):504]. Otolaryngol Head Neck Surg 2014;150(1 suppl):S1–24.
50. Marchisio P, Espositio S, Bianchini S. Efficacy of injectable trivalent virosomal adjuvanted inactivated influenza vaccine in preventing acute otitis media in children with recurrent complicated or noncomplicated acute otitis media. Pediatr Infect Dis J 2009;28(10):855–9.

Vestibular Disorders

Prabhat K. Pokhrel, MS, MD, PhD*, Rose Hall, DO,
Melanie Pendergrass, DO, Jasmine Kaur, MD

KEYWORDS

- Vestibular disorders • Vestibular migraine • Vestibular neuritis
- Ménière's disease or endolymphatic hydrops • Benign paroxysmal positional vertigo

KEY POINTS

- Vestibular disorder is a dysfunction in the balance system of the body either due to malfunctioning of the inner ear or due to central nervous system dysfunction or both.
- Vestibular neuritis is defined by an acute onset of vertigo for 24 hours or more without hearing loss.
- Typical symptoms of vestibular dysfunctions include vertigo, vestibulo-visual symptoms, postural symptoms, and tinnitus.
- Common types of acute peripheral vestibular dysfunction include benign paroxysmal positional vertigo, vestibular neuritis, Ménière's disease, and vestibular migraine.
- Demyelinating disease such as multiple sclerosis and ototoxic medications can also cause vestibular symptoms.

INTRODUCTION TO VESTIBULAR DISORDERS

The term vestibular disorder (VD) means the condition is related to vestibular structure (peripheral and central) or its mechanism. On the other hand, vestibular symptoms or dysfunctions are broader terminologies and include symptoms not related or partially related to vestibular apparatus or mechanism.[1] Vestibular system consists of (a) peripheral vestibular structures located in the inner ear (balance system), which include the utricle, the saccule, and 3 semicircular canals (lateral, superior, and posterior) and (b) brainstem and cerebellum (processing centers). Together with visual and somatosensory systems, structures of the inner ear fire signals to the central nervous system (CNS) to maintain balance, and orient head and body in space.[2] If a lesion is in the inner ear, it is classified as peripheral vestibular disorder, and if a lesion is in the CNS, it is known as central vestibular disorder.

This review article focuses mainly on the diagnosis and management of the common peripheral VD such as benign paroxysmal positional vertigo (BPPV), Ménière's disease, vestibular migraine, and vestibular neuritis.

Department of Family Medicine, McLaren Flint, G-3230 Beecher Road, Suite 1, Flint, MI 48532, USA
* Corresponding author.
E-mail address: prabhat.pokhrel@mclaren.org

Prim Care Clin Office Pract 52 (2025) 15–25
https://doi.org/10.1016/j.pop.2024.09.004   **primarycare.theclinics.com**

Both central and peripheral VD can be acute (up to 2 weeks), subacute (up to 3 months), and chronic (more than 3 months). Detailed history and physical examinations aid in identifying the type of VD, which is critical in managing different types of VDs. Estimated 33 million adults and 3.5 million children and adolescents in the United States are affected by VD.[3]

Etiology of vestibular disorders is multifactorial. Depending on the etiology of vestibular disorder, symptoms may vary.[4] Symptoms of central and peripheral vestibular disorders usually present acutely and include vertigo, tinnitus, nausea, vomiting, unsteady gait, fall, and nystagmus.[3,5] Symptoms of acute vestibular disorders may last from a week to few months and may become chronic. For example, unilateral vestibular nerve pathology may cause nystagmus, dizziness, gait disturbance, and sensation of dizziness with head movement. Nystagmus and dizziness in unilateral vestibular nerve impairment may last 1 to 2 weeks, but unsteady gait may last weeks to months.[6] More than 1 vestibular disorder may occur simultaneously in some patients. Vestibular migraine may co-exist with BPPV, and Ménière's disease may co-exist with vestibular migraine. In general, patient education and appropriate symptomatic treatments may be enough in managing vestibular disorders of peripheral origin, whereas treatments for the central vestibular disorders are disease-specific. Management of peripheral VDs includes pharmacotherapy, vestibular rehabilitation, psychotherapy, and rarely surgery. Kamo and colleagues have reported that early vestibular rehabilitation improved several measured outcomes in patients with acute vestibular disorders.[6] Often pharmacotherapy is started without a definite diagnosis for the symptomatic treatment of vestibular disorders.[7] Because of the broad differential diagnoses of VDs, a multidisciplinary approach may be needed when managing patients with VDs. Vestibular disorders if not managed properly can increase risk of fall, loss of workdays, and may adversely affect quality of life of the patients.

VERTIGO, DIZZINESS, AND TINNITUS

Vertigo, dizziness, and tinnitus are frequent causes of primary care, emergency room visits, and referral to a consultation. The International Classification of Vestibular Disorders of the Bárány Society defines vertigo as a sensation of self-motion when no self-motion is occurring or the sensation of distorted self-motion during an otherwise normal head movement. It defines dizziness as a sensation of altered spatial orientation without the feeling of false motion. According to this classification, vertigo is considered a separate entity but not a type of dizziness.[8] Vertigo and dizziness are common symptoms of vestibular disorders. Both can be spontaneous without obvious triggers or triggered with an identifiable cause. Common triggers of vertigo are position of the head, head movement, sound, visual (seeing objects in motion), straining (Valsalva maneuver), and orthostatic.[8] Peripheral vertigo is most common in BPPV followed by Ménière disease and vestibular neuritis.[9] Tinnitus is a perceived sound in the absence of an internal or external source. Tinnitus is usually benign in nature. While there is no universal cause of tinnitus, risk factors include sensory neural hearing loss, loud noise exposure, trauma, infection, and medications. Evaluation begins with a history and physical, followed by audiology evaluation. There is no cure for tinnitus, however, there are treatment strategies that can be utilized to alleviate symptoms and improve quality of life. These treatment options encompass directed attention and habituation through various methods including, but not limited to, tinnitus retraining therapy, cognitive behavior therapy, tinnitus activities treatment, and progressive tinnitus management.[10]

BENIGN PAROXYSMAL POSITIONAL VERTIGO

As the name suggests, BPPV is characterized by a brief, spinning sensations elicited by a change in the position of the head and lasts few seconds. According to the American Academy of Otolaryngology-Head and Neck Surgery Foundation Clinical Practice Guideline, diagnostic criteria for posterior canal BPPV are repeated episodes of vertigo with changes in head position and vertigo associated with nystagmus that is provoked by the Dix-Hallpike test. It is important to keep in mind that there is a latency period of about 60 seconds between the completion of the Dix-Hallpike test and the onset of vertigo and nystagmus.[11] Besides being the most common cause of vertigo, BPPV is also the most common vestibular disorder in adults. About 42% of patients with vertigo are diagnosed with BPPV. It is more common in females than in males (2:1) and with a peak onset between 50 and 70 years of age.[12] Vertigo in patients with BPPV is brief, lasting between 30 and 60 seconds, and triggered by a change in the position of the head relative to gravity, such as tilting one's head back, rolling over in bed, or going down to or getting up from the bed. In addition to vertigo, BPPV may lead to nausea, vomiting, decreased work performance, depression, and fall which could be partly due to a reported association of BPPV with osteopenia or osteoporosis.[12] BPPV is not associated with hearing loss.[13] Often, BPPV is underdiagnosed or even misdiagnosed.

Underlying pathophysiology of BPPV is a free-floating otoconia (canalithiasis) entering one of the semi-circular canals, mainly posterior semicircular canal (up to 90% of all cases), followed by horizontal and then anterior semi-circular canal. Detached otoconia from the utricular otolith, now reside in one of the semi-circular canals, and move to a new position with the movement of the head, creating a false sensation of rotation.[14,15]

BPPV usually is unilateral, but bilateral and multiple canals BPPV have been reported but it is rare. Most cases of BPPV are idiopathic. Head injury, vestibular neuritis, and Ménière's disease have been reported to lead to BPPV. Prognosis of BPPV is usually very good with many cases going into spontaneous remission within 12 weeks, especially if the horizontal semi-circular canal is involved. Although, BPPV may last a few weeks, but each episode of BPPV lasts only for a few seconds.

Differential diagnosis of BPPV includes stroke, vestibular neuritis, vestibular migraine, Ménière's disease, and labyrinthitis. A thorough history, physical examination, medication review, and additional appropriate testing may help identify the underlying cause of acute episodic vertigo. According to BPPV guideline evidence-based statements, "Clinician should diagnose posterior semicircular canal BPPV when vertigo associated with nystagmus is provoked by the Dix-Hallpike maneuver, performed by bringing the patient from an upright to supine position with the head turned 45° to one side and neck extended 20°" (Strong recommendation). The Dix-Hallpike maneuver is considered the gold standard test to diagnose posterior canal BPPV and should be performed bilaterally to determine which side is involved and to find out whether it is unilateral or bilateral. Patients with certain co-morbid conditions such as cervical stenosis, severe rheumatoid arthritis, morbid obesity, and others are at increased risk of complications from the Dix-Hallpike maneuver.[11] Dix-Hallpike maneuvers should not be performed if a patient has neurologic signs or symptoms, and a patient is dizzy when still. Patients with a high index of suspicion for BPPV in whom Dix-Hallpike test is negative, should be tested for horizontal or lateral semi-circular canal BPPV using supine roll test.[11] The technique to perform supine roll test can be viewed at https://www.youtube.com/watch?v=U3SGJfjwJaw.

TREATMENT OF POSTERIOR CANAL BENIGN PAROXYSMAL POSITIONAL VERTIGO

Although spontaneous resolution of BPPV is possible within few weeks from the time of onset, recovery can be expedited using particle repositioning maneuver (PRM).[15] Epley (canalith repositing procedure) and Semont (liberatory) maneuvers are the 2 most used PRM in clinical practice and can be performed in the office. Both techniques are therapeutic may eliminate vertigo due to BPPV. Number of times a patient may have to undergo PRM varies from 1 to many with no reported optimal numbers. Techniques to perform Dix-Hallpike maneuver and Semont maneuver are shown in **Figs 1** and **2**, respectively. The Semont maneuver can be substituted with Epley's maneuver.[16] Before performing any of these maneuvers, patients should be made aware of possible worsening of vertigo, nausea, and vomiting. Anti-emetic medications may be prescribed in some patients before the procedure based on shared decision-making.

Steps to perform Epley's maneuver can be viewed at https://www.youtube.com/watch?v=LxD-lgqix-s.

Vestibular rehabilitation (VR) which is performed by a trained physical therapist can be used as initial therapy for BPPV. Patients with persistent BPPV should be re-evaluated for alternative diagnosis as central nervous system disorder may co-exist with BPPV. Surgical treatment for BPPV is rare and needed for cases refractory to PRM or VR. It is not recommended to routinely prescribe vestibular suppressant therapy like antihistamines or benzodiazepine.[11]

VESTIBULAR NEURITIS OR VESTIBULAR NEURONITIS

Vestibular neuritis (VN) is characterized by an acute onset of spinning vertigo lasting at least for 24 hours without hearing loss and central neurologic signs. Most patients with VN are between 40 and 70 years of age. Rotational vertigo in VN peaks on the first day

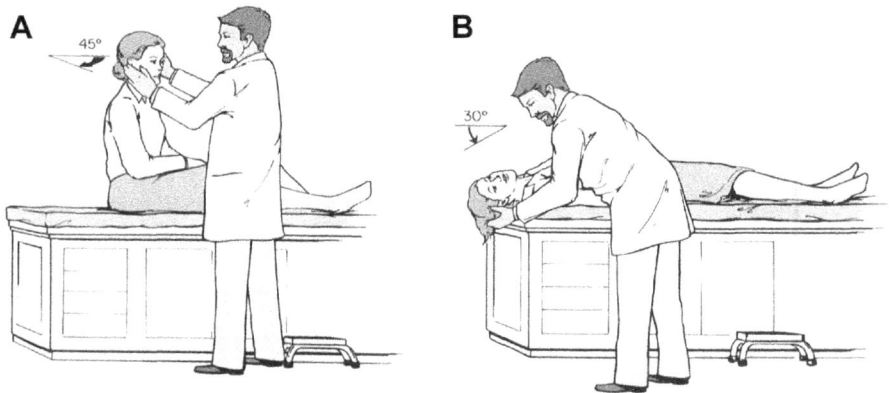

Fig. 1. Dix-Hallpike maneuver (right ear). The patient is seated and positioned so that the patient's head will extend over the top edge of the table when supine. The head is turned 45° toward the ear being tested (*position A*). The patient is quickly lowered into the supine position with the head extending about 30° below the horizontal (*position B*). The patient's head is held in this position and the examiner observes the patient's eyes for nystagmus. To complete the maneuver, the patient is returned to the seated position (position A) and the eyes are observed for the reverasal nystagmus, in this case, a fast-phase clockwise nystagmus. (*From* Parnes LS, Agrawal SK, Atlas J. Diagnosis and management of benign paroxysmal positional vertigo (BPPV). CMAJ 2003; 169(7): 681-93 with permission.)

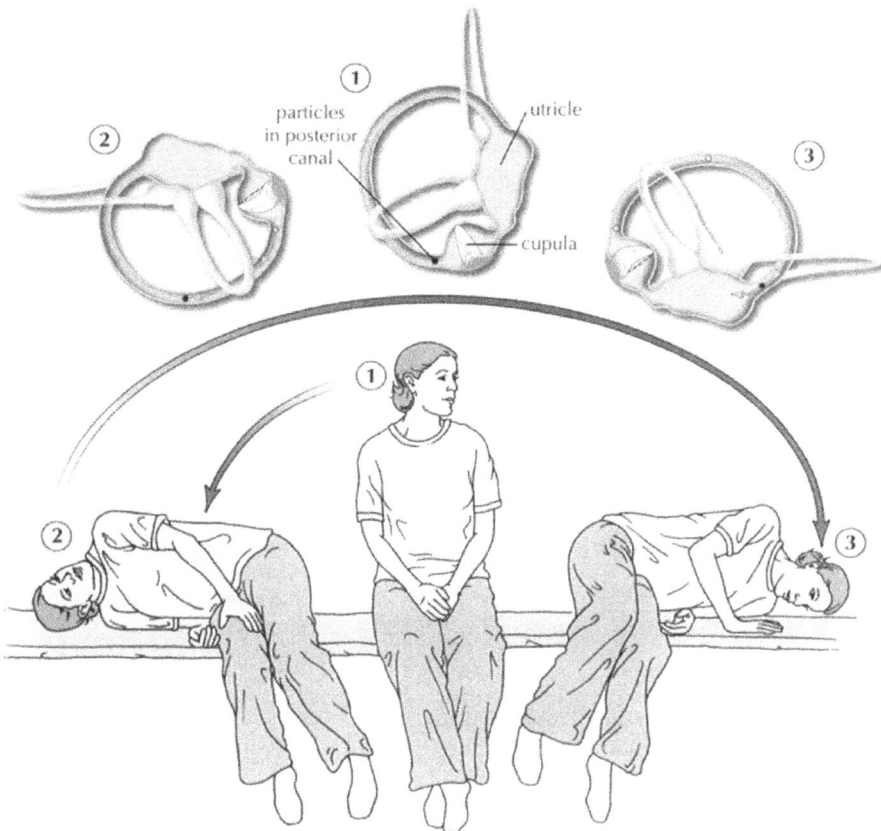

Fig. 2. Liberatory maneuver of Semont (right ear). The top panel shows the effect of the maneuver on the labyrinth as viewed from the front and the induced movement of the canaliths. This maneuver relies on inertia, so that the transition from position 2 to 3 must be made very quickly. (*From* Parnes LS, Agrawal SK, Atlas J. Diagnosis and management of benign paroxysmal positional vertigo (BPPV). CMAJ 2003; 169(7): 681-93 with permission.)

and patients usually prefer lying down on the side with the healthy ear over the pillow, which may improve over the period of few days.[17]

Etiology of VN is unknown. Viral infections (coronavirus disease 2019 [COVID-19] and human simplex virus type 1) and adenoviral vector-based COVID-19 vaccines,[18,19] autoimmune disorder affecting vestibular nerve, and vestibular artery ischemia are proposed etiologies of VN. Secondary BPPV could be a result of VN, although the exact relationship between the 2 is unknown.[20]

DIAGNOSIS OF VESTIBULAR NEURONITIS

Sustained rotational vertigo in VN may be preceded by spells of episodic vertigo few days prior. Vertigo is often accompanied by spontaneous peripheral horizontal vestibular nystagmus, nausea with or without vomiting, and ataxia. Ataxia in VN is manifested as body tilting to the diseased side and may result in fall. Tinnitus, ear pain, diplopia, recent trauma, and signs and symptoms of stroke are absent in VN, and if present diagnoses other than VN, such as Ménière's disease, herpes zoster infection, infarction of the cerebellum, and brainstem should be considered.[21]

Tests helpful in diagnosing VN include head impulse test, bi-thermal caloric test, and vestibular-evoked myogenic potential test. The head impulse test (sensitivity ranges from 0% to 100% with median sensitivity 41%% and specificity ranged between 56% and 100% (median 94%)[22] is an easy test to perform in a primary care office. To perform this test, the patient in a seated position fixed his eyes on examiner's nose and the examiner focused his or her eyes on the patient's eye. The examiner holds patient's head on both sides and moves the head to the affected side and back with a small-amplitude, high-accelerated motion. Same maneuver is repeated to the other "unaffected side." Examiner should look for corrective rapid eye movement (saccades) and if present indicates peripheral vestibular lesion.[23] If inconclusive, referral to a subspecialist for possible bi-thermal caloric test and vestibular-evoked myogenic potential tests is appropriate after going through the algorithm steps as outline by Rogers and colleagues (2023) and Muncie and colleagues[24,25]

Treatment of VN can be categorized into (a) symptomatic therapy, (b) specific drug therapy, and (c) vestibular rehabilitation. Symptomatic therapy involves supportive care, anti-emetics (ondansetron, metoclopramide), and vestibular suppressants (dimenhydrinate, meclizine, scopolamine). Specific drug therapy is controversial and includes methylprednisolone, antiviral, and vasodilator therapy. Vestibular rehabilitation therapy is geared toward improving vertigo, gaze, and postural stability and improving the quality of life. With appropriate therapeutic interventions, up to 70% of patients with VN recover completely with a recurrence rate up to 11%.[24]

Vestibular Migraine

Vestibular migraine (VM) affects 1% to 2.7% of the population and is the most common cause of non-positional vertigo.[26] Patients diagnosed with VM have recurrent episodes of moderate to severe vestibular symptoms associated with photophobia, phonophobia, visual aura, with or without migraine like headaches.[27,28] In 2012, the International Classification of Headache Disorders and the International Classification of Vestibular Disorder Barany Society created criteria for the classification of VM which help aid in the diagnosis since there is no gold standard diagnostic testing.[26] It may be difficult to diagnose VM from other vestibular disorders, especially in its chronic form. Diagnostic criteria for VM are listed in **Box 1**.[29,30] If diagnosis is unclear, performing audiometry and/or vestibular testing should be considered to help rule out Ménière's disease, benign positional vertigo, and other causes.[27] An MRI of the brain may be indicated if tansient ischemic attack (TIA) or stroke is suspected.

The exact pathophysiology of VM is not known and is thought to be a multifactorial interaction between the trigeminal and vestibular systems.[27] It has been hypothesized that vasospasms during migraines lead to hypoperfusion of the inner ear resulting in vertigo and sudden sensory neuronal hearing loss and tinnitus.[26,31] Another potential mechanism reported is that there is a release of pro-inflammatory neuropeptide substance P and calcitonin gene-related peptide from the activation of the trigeminovascular system leading to signs and symptoms of VM.[26]

Treatment of VM can be broken down to abortive treatment and preventative treatment. For all patients who are diagnosed with VM, it is recommended to discuss appropriate healthy lifestyle changes regarding sleep hygiene, physical exercise, stress management, potential dietary triggers, and regular meals.[27,28] Abortive treatment focuses on treating the headache, vertigo, and nausea symptoms with simple analgesics, non-steroidal anti-inflammatory drugs, triptans, and medications that modulate the vestibular symptoms like cyclizine, prochlorperazine, dimenhydrinate,

> **Box 1**
> **Diagnostic criteria for vestibular migraine based on the International Classification of Headache Disorders, 3rd edition**
>
> Vestibular migraine (International Classification of Headache Disorders [ICHD-3] and International Classification of Vestibular Disorders (ICVD)
> A. At least 5 episodes fulfilling criteria C and D,
> B. A current or past history of migraine without aura or migraine with aura,
> C. Vestibular symptoms of moderate or severe intensity, lasting between 5 minutes and 72 hours,
> D. At least 50% of episodes are associated with at least one of the following 3 migrainous features:
>   1. Headache with at least 2 of the following 4 characteristics:
>   a. Unilateral location
>   b. Pulsating quality
>   c. Moderate or severe intensity
>   d. Aggravation by routine physical activity
>   2. Photophobia and phonophobia
>   3. Visual aura
> E. Not better accounted for by another ICHD-3 diagnosis or by another vestibular disorder
>
> Probable vestibular migraine (ICVD)
> A. At least 5 episodes with vestibular symptoms of moderate or severe intensity, lasting 5 min to 72 hours,
> B. Only one of the criteria B and D for vestibular migraine is fulfilled (migraine history or migraine features during the episode),
> C. Not better accounted for another vestibular or ICHD diagnosis.
>
> *From* Headache Classification Committee of the International Headache Society (IHS). The International Classification of Headache Disorders, 3rd edition. Cephalalgia 2018; 38: 1–211) and Lempert T, Olesen J, Furman J, et al. Vestibular migraine: Diagnostic criteria (Update). J Vestib Res 2022; 32:1–6.

meclizine, and cinnarizine. Abortive treatment should be used less than 10 days per month. For preventative treatment of VM, the most efficacious medications with the lowest rates of serious side effects are amitriptyline and nortriptyline, propranolol, metoprolol, and verapamil.[27,28] Other medications reported to be efficacious but have increased risk of serious unwanted effects are topiramate, sodium valproate, venlafaxine, lamotrigine, candesartan, supplements (riboflavin/coenzyme Q 10/magnesium), and botulism toxin A, which have limited efficacy evidence but could be considered if there is failure with the previously mentioned treatments. For patients who do not respond to traditional treatment, or those who want to pursue nonpharmacological approaches, vestibular rehabilitation may be considered.[27]

MÉNIÈRE'S DISEASE

Ménière's Disease (MD) is an inner ear disorder that mostly affects people aged 30 to 60 years of age and presents as spontaneous recurrent vertigo usually rotational, fluctuating sensorineural hearing loss, fullness, and tinnitus in the affected ear, mostly unilateral. Pathophysiology of the MD is not completely understood. It is partly thought to be due to accumulation of endolymphatic fluid in cochlea and vestibular organ leading to endolymphatic hydrops.[32,33]

Symptoms of MD may last decades and could significantly impact patient's quality of life. The etiology of MD is multifactorial and has been associated with allergies, autoimmune diseases, infection, and trauma.[34,35] Several studies have reported higher prevalence of migraine with MD.[36]

The American Academy of Otolaryngology-Head and Neck Surgery, the European Academy of Otology and Neurotology, the Japan Society for Equilibrium Research, and the Korean Balance Society have recommended the following clinical diagnostic criteria for MD.[33]

DEFINITIVE DIAGNOSTIC CRITERIA:

- Two or more spontaneous attacks of vertigo, each lasting 20 minutes to 12 hours,[37]
- Audiometrically documented fluctuating low to midfrequency sensorineural hearing loss in the affected ear on at least 1 occasion before, during, or after 1 of the episodes of vertigo,
- Fluctuating aural symptoms (hearing loss, tinnitus, or fullness) in the affected ear,
- Other causes excluded by other tests.

PROBABLE DIAGNOSTIC CRITERIA

- At least 2 episodes of vertigo or dizziness lasting 20 minutes to 24 hours,
- Fluctuating aural symptoms (hearing loss, tinnitus, or fullness) in the affected ear,
- Other causes excluded by other tests.

Audiometry, vestibular function tests, gadolinium-enhanced MRI may aid in diagnosing MD.[33]

In primary care offices, audiometry together with Weber and Rinne Tests may help different conductive and sensorineural or missed hearing loss. Weber and Rinne tests are useful only identifying unilateral hearing loss. Procedure on how to perform these tests and how to interpret the results can be found at https://www.youtube.com/watch?v=Y8jHmEEFI5Y. Pay attention to the position of the 2 arms of the tuning fork during Rinne's test. In fact, audiometric evaluation is mandatory in all patients with MD.

Several symptomatic treatment strategies exist for MD but none of them cure the disease. Lifestyle modification such as restriction of salt (below 2300 mg a day), caffeine, tobacco, alcohol intake, and reduction of stress, anxiety, and high quality of sleep are the first-line treatments and may help reduce the MD attacks.[32] Thiazide diuretics (hydrochlorothiazide or chlorthalidone) are the first-line pharmacotherapy to reduce the frequency and severity of the symptoms but not hearing loss. Intratympanic steroid injections (dexamethasone or methylprednisolone) may reduce frequency of vertigo attacks and preserve auditory function.[38] Intratympanic gentamicin injection has some evidence to attenuate symptoms of MD but it is also ototoxic and is used for the treatment in refractory MD.[39] Low-dose gentamicin therapy (40 mg/mL or lower) may help patients strike a balance between vertigo control and preservation of hearing.[40] The first generation antihistamines (meclizine, dimenhydrinate) can be used for milder attacks; anti-dopaminergic drugs (metoclopramide, promethazine, and prochlorperazine) and serotonin antagonists such as ondansetron are used for severe nausea and vomiting.[41] Surgical treatment like endolymphatic sac surgery, labyrinthectomy, and vestibular neurectomy are additional options and recommended if pharmacotherapy is ineffective.[39]

Prognosis of MD is progressive with unpredictable fluctuations. Frequency of vertigo decreases over the years but at a cost of hearing loss. Due to the paucity of high-quality randomized controlled trials, clinically it is hard to conclude whether attenuations of the symptoms are a part of the natural course of the MD or effects of treatment or both.[42]

CLINICS CARE POINTS

- Vestibular disease is common and an important clinical entity for health care providers to understand since it does affect quality of life of patients.
- Peripheral vestibular disorders must be differentiated from the central vestibular disorder, such as ischemic stroke since treatments are different.
- Assessing type of hearing loss with an audiogram, and Weber and Rinne tests may aid in the diagnosis of vestibular disorder.

DISCLOSURE

The authors have nothing to disclose.

REFERENCES

1. Bisdorff A, Von Brevern M, Lempert T, et al. Classification of vestibular symptoms: towards an international classification of vestibular disorders. J Vestib Res 2009; 19:1–13.
2. Hughes A. Vestibular and central nervous system, anatomy. In: Kountakis SE, editor. Encyclopedia of Otolaryngology, head and neck surgery. Berlin: Springer; 2013. p. 3014–6.
3. Sayegh MA, Banaag A, Korona-Bailey J, et al. The burden of vestibular disorders among military health system(MHS) beneficiaries, fiscal years 2018–2019. PLoS One 2023;18:1–9.
4. Xing Y, Si L, Zhang W, et al. Etiologic distribution of dizziness/vertigo in a neurological outpatient clinic according to the criteria of the international classification of vestibular disorders: a single-center study. J Neurol 2024. https://doi.org/10.1007/s00415-023-12166-3/. Accessed March 01, 2024.
5. Donovan J, De Silva L, Cox H, et al. Vestibular dysfunction in people who fall: a systematic review and meta-analysis of prevalence and associated factors. Clin Rehabil 2023;37:1229–47.
6. Kamo T, Ogihara H, Azami M, et al. Effects of early vestibular rehabilitation in patients with acute vestibular disorder: a systematic review and meta-analysis. Otol Neurotol 2023;44:e641–7.
7. Aran MB, Ocak E, Buyukatalay ZA, et al. Medical treatment approaches in vestibular disorders: a descriptive cross-sectional study. J Ear, Nose, Throat Head Neck Surgery 2023;31:157–61.
8. Fife TD. Approach to the history and evaluation of vertigo and dizziness. Continuum 2021;27:306–29.
9. Strupp M, Magnusson M. Acute unilateral vestibulopathy. Neurol Clin 2015;33: 669–85.
10. Henry JA. Directed attention and habituation: two concepts critical to tinnitus management. Am J Audiol 2023;32:274–81.
11. Bhattacharyya N, Baugh RF, Orvidas L, et al. Clinical practice guideline: benign paroxysmal positional vertigo. Otolaryngol Head Neck Surg 2008;139(Suppl 4):S47–81.
12. von Brevern M, Radtke A, Lezius F, et al. Epidemiology of benign paroxysmal positional vertigo: a population-based study. J Neurol Neurosurg Psychiatry 2007; 78:710–5.
13. Lopez-Escamez JA, Gamiz MJ, Fernandez-Perez A, et al. Long-term outcome and health-related quality of life in benign paroxysmal positional vertigo. Eur Arch Oto-Rhino-Laryngol 2005;262:507–11.

14. Furman JM, Cass SP. Benign paroxysmal positional vertigo. N Engl J Med 1999; 341:1590–6.
15. Kim J, Zee DS. Benign paroxysmal positional vertigo. N Engl J Med 2014;1138–47.
16. Parnes LS, Agrawal SK, Atlas J. Diagnosis and management of benign paroxysmal positional vertigo (BPPV). CMAJ (Can Med Assoc J) 2003;169:681–93.
17. Le TN, Westerberg BD, Lea J. Vestibular neuritis: recent advances in etiology, diagnostic evaluation, and treatment. Adv Oto-Rhino-Laryngol 2019;82:87–92.
18. Shahali H, Hamidi Farahani R, Hazrati P. Acute vestibular neuritis: a rare complication after the adenoviral vector-based COVID-19 vaccine. J Neurovirol 2022; 28:609–15. https://doi.org/10.1007/s13365-022-01087-y. Accessed April 17, 2024.
19. Jeong J, Nam Y, Oh J, et al. Monthly and seasonal variations in vestibular neuritis. Medicine (United States) 2022;101(26):E29787. https://doi.org/10.1097/MD.0000000000029787. Accessed April 17, 2024.
20. Bae CH, Na HG, Choi YS. Current diagnosis and treatment of vestibular neuritis: a narrative review. Journal of Yeungnam Medical Science 2022;39:81–8. https://doi.org/10.12701/yujm.2021.01228. Accessed April 17, 2024.
21. Strupp M, Bisdorff A, Furman J, et al. Acute unilateral vestibulopathy/vestibular neuritis: diagnostic criteria. J Vestib Res 2022;32:389–406.
22. Walther LE, Löhler J, Agrawal Y, et al. Evaluating the diagnostic accuracy of the head-impulse test: a scoping review. JAMA Otolaryngol Head Neck Surg 2019; 145(6):550–60. https://doi.org/10.1001/jamaoto.2019.0243.
23. Choi KD, Oh SY, Kim JS. Head thrust test. Ann Clin Neurophysiol 2006;8:1–5.
24. Rogers TS, Noel MA, Garcia B. Dizziness: evaluation and management. Am Fam Physician 2023;107:514–23.
25. Kim JS. When the room is spinning: experience of vestibular neuritis by a neurotologist. Front Neurol 2020;11:157. https://doi.org/10.3389/fneur.2020.00157. Accessed May 13, 2024.
26. Smyth D, Britton Z, Murdin L, et al. Vestibular migraine treatment: a comprehensive practical review. Brain 2022;145:3741–54.
27. Mallampalli MP, Rizk HG, Kheradmand A, et al. Care gaps and recommendations in vestibular migraine: an expert panel summit. Front Neurol 2022;12:2021. https://doi.org/10.3389/fneur.2021.812678.
28. Beh Shin C, Vestibular Migraine MD. How to sort it out and what to do about it. J Neuro Ophthalmol 2019;39:208–19.
29. Headache Classification Committee of the International Headache Society (IHS). The International classification of headache disorders, 3rd ed. Cephalalgia 2018; 38:1–211.
30. Lempert T, Olesen J, Furman J, et al. Vestibular migraine: diagnostic criteria (Update). J Vestib Res 2022;32:1–6.
31. Abouzari M, Tawk K, Lee D, et al. Migrainous vertigo, tinnitus, and ear symptoms and alternatives. Otolaryngol Clin 2022;55:1017–33. Available at: https://escholarship.org/uc/item/9mk2p14c. Accessed May 25, 2024.
32. Oğuz E, Cebeci A, Geçici CR. The relationship between nutrition and Ménière's disease. Auris Nasus Larynx 2021;48:803–8.
33. Perez-Carpena P, Lopez-Escamez J. Current understanding and clinical management of ménière's disease: a systematic review. Semin Neurol 2020;40:138–50.
34. Lopez-Escamez JA, Vela J, Frejo L. Immune-related disorders associated with ménière's disease: a systematic review and meta-analysis. Otolaryngol Head Neck Surg 2023;169:1122–31.

35. Mohseni-Dargah M, Falahati Z, Pastras C, et al. Ménière's disease: pathogenesis, treatments, and emerging approaches for an idiopathic bioenvironmental disorder. Environ Res 2023;238(Part 1):116972. https://doi.org/10.1016/j.envres.2023.116972. Accessed April 20, 2024.
36. Ray J, Carr SD, Popli G, et al. An epidemiological study to investigate the relationship between Ménière's disease and migraine. Clin Otolaryngol 2016;41:707–10.
37. Basura G, Kerber K, Adams M, et al. Clinical practice guideline: Ménière's disease executive summary. Otolaryngology 2020;162:415–34.
38. Hoskin JL. Ménière's disease: new guidelines, subtypes, imaging, and more. Curr Opin Neurol 2022;35:90–7.
39. Liu Y, Yang J, Duan M. Current status on researches of Ménière's disease: a review. Acta Otolaryngol 2020;140:808–12.
40. Hao W, Yu H, Li H. Effects of intratympanic gentamicin and intratympanic glucocorticoids in Ménière's disease: a network meta-analysis. J Neurol 2022;269:72–86.
41. Espinosa-Sanchez JM, Lopez-Escamez JA. The pharmacological management of vertigo in Meniere disease. Expet Opin Pharmacother 2020;21:1753–63.
42. Wright T. Ménière's disease. In: The senses: a comprehenisve reference. 2015. https://doi.org/10.1016/B978-012370880-9.00015-3. Available at: https://escholarship.org/uc/item/6xr7p2hj. Accessed April 29, 2024.

Tonsillitis

Van Tuong Ngoc Nguyen, DO, FAAFP, DipABOM[a,b,c,]*,
Larry Ngo, MD, FAAP[b,d], Erica Stratton, MD[a,b,c], Daniel Arriola, MD[a,b]

KEYWORDS

- Strep throat • Tonsillitis • Pharyngitis • Sore throat
- Group A beta-hemolytic Streptococcus

KEY POINTS

- Acute tonsillitis most commonly affects the pediatric population, presenting with sore throat and difficulty swallowing.
- The modified Centor criteria can guide treatment plan for diagnostic testing and/or empiric treatment of group A beta-hemolytic Streptococcus.
- Acute tonsillitis secondary to group A beta-hemolytic Streptococcus should be treated with appropriate antibiotics to prevent complications such as acute rheumatic fever.
- Anti-streptolysin O titers should not be ordered for acute tonsillitis as it is only used in the diagnosis of acute rheumatic fever, not acute tonsillitis.
- Systemic corticosteroids are not recommended routinely for acute tonsillitis.

INTRODUCTION

The purpose of this article is to review the currently available material pertaining to tonsillitis. It is a common illness that affects patients of all age ranges but more commonly in the young. Clinical presentation is highly variable and similar symptoms are noted in viral and bacterial tonsillitis. This article focuses on the clinical presentation, diagnosis, and management of this important disease to mitigate the risk of significant morbidity and mortality such as acute rheumatic fever (ARF).

BACKGROUND

Pharyngitis is a common diagnosis that causes patients to seek care from their primary care physician. It accounts for almost 2% of primary care ambulatory care visits each year.[1] Of these, approximately 5% are due to group A beta-hemolytic

[a] Family Medicine Residency, Loma Linda University Medical Center-Murrieta, Murrieta, CA, USA; [b] Loma Linda University School of Medicine, Loma Linda, CA, USA; [c] Department of Family Medicine, Loma Linda University Health, Loma Linda, CA, USA; [d] Department of Pediatrics, Loma Linda University Children's Hospital, Loma Linda, CA, USA
* Corresponding author. Department of Family Medicine, Loma Linda University Health, 28062 Baxter Road, Murrieta, CA 92563.
E-mail address: vatnguyen@llu.edu

Prim Care Clin Office Pract 52 (2025) 27–35
https://doi.org/10.1016/j.pop.2024.09.005
0095-4543/25/© 2024 Elsevier Inc. All rights reserved, including those for text and data mining, AI training, and similar technologies.
primarycare.theclinics.com

streptococci or *Streptococcus pyogenes* tonsillitis.[2] This review article will focus on tonsillitis.

Tonsillitis is most commonly due to a viral infection and thus self-limiting. Up to 15% of tonsillitis in adults, and 30% in the pediatric population, however, are due to a bacterial etiology.[3] The most common bacterial cause of tonsillitis is infection by group A beta-hemolytic streptococcus, commonly known as strep throat.[3–5]

PATHOPHYSIOLOGY

Tonsils are lymphoid tissues located in the nasopharynx and oral pharynx. This includes the pharyngeal, tubal, lingual, and palatine tonsils. These tissues play an important role in the immune system in exposure to virus or bacteria to the respiratory and gastrointestinal tract. They contain B cells, microfold M cells, T cells, and macrophages that are involved in the presentation, recognition, and response to infectious antigens.[6,7]

CAUSES

Tonsillitis is caused by viral or bacterial infection of the naso-oro-pharynx. The nasopharynx has hundreds of viruses and bacteria, making it difficult to determine the pathologic etiology of tonsillitis. However, it is suggested that viral infections are implicated in 70% to 95% of all cases.[2] The most common viruses causing acute tonsillitis in the pediatric population are adenovirus, influenza, parainfluenza, Epstein–Barr Virus, human herpes virus 3, and enteroviruses.[8] In adults, almost 50% of cases are due to rhinovirus or coronavirus.[8]

The most common viral and bacterial etiologies are listed in **Table 1**.[9,10]

RISK FACTORS

Patients who are at risk for development of tonsillitis include those who have high exposure to respiratory and viral infections. These populations include school-aged children from 5 to 15 years old and those who work with or have frequent contact with children. Patients who are immunocompromised are also at higher risk for tonsillitis.[11]

CLINICAL SYMPTOMS AND SIGNS

Tonsillitis is a clinical diagnosis that is rooted in a thorough history and physical examination of the nasopharynx and oropharynx. Patients will often present with a constellation of symptoms including fever, tonsillar exudates, cough, anorexia, congestion,

Table 1 Etiologies of acute tonsillitis[9,10]	
Viral Etiologies	**Bacterial Etiologies**
Adenovirus	*Group A beta-hemolytic streptococcus*
Coronavirus	*Staphylococcus aureus*
Epstein–Barr virus	*Streptococcus pneumoniae*
Cytomegalovirus	*Haemophilus influenza*
Hepatitis A	*Corynebacterium diphtheriae*
Herpes simplex virus	Syphilis
Human immunodeficiency virus	Chlamydia
Influenza	Gonorrhea
Respiratory syncytial virus	Tuberculosis
Rhinovirus	

and/or tender cervical lymphadenopathy. Less commonly, patients with tonsillitis will present without upper respiratory symptoms. Associated symptoms include palatal petechiae, strawberry tongue, erythematous or edematous uvula, or rash. Headaches, myalgias, nausea and vomiting, and abdominal pain are not common in tonsillitis.[12]

Signs and symptoms associated with more severe cases of tonsillitis include dysphagia and/or odynophagia due to tonsillar swelling.[12] Enlargement of the tonsils may also cause narrowing of the posterior oropharynx, leading to hoarseness, and affect the patient's ability to maintain and protect the airway. Uvula deviation may be indicative of a tonsillar abscess.[10] Other symptoms that warrant more urgent evaluation in the emergency department are trismus, muffled voice, uvula deviation, drooling, or unilateral facial swelling.

Table 2 reviews the common associated signs and symptoms of viral versus bacterial tonsillitis.[10]

DIAGNOSIS

Tonsillitis is a clinical diagnosis. Determining viral versus bacterial etiology is of utmost importance for antibiotic stewardship.

Clinical Diagnosis

Obtaining a thorough history and physical is essential in the diagnosis of tonsillitis. History should focus on the presence of fever and absence of cough. And, the physical examination should assess for tonsillar enlargement, tonsillar exudate, and tender cervical lymphadenopathy. It is these history and physical components and patient age that comprise the modified Centor (McIsaac) score; one point is assigned to each of these components. The Centor score risk stratifies patients with possible group A beta-hemolytic streptococcus (GAS) tonsillitis. Scores of 1 or less are low risk for GAS tonsillitis and do not require any further testing. If there is high clinical suspicion for GAS tonsillitis and a Centor score of 2 or 3, further testing can with point-of-care testing or throat culture should be considered. Scores of 4 or more should be treated with empiric antibiotics regardless of point-of-care testing and a throat culture obtained. The modified Centor score was created to estimate the probability of tonsillitis to be secondary to streptococcus; it was meant to provide support for immediate treatment of bacterial tonsillitis while being judicious in the use of antibiotics.[2,3,13]

Laboratory Testing

Testing for GAS tonsillitis is not recommended for patients aged less than 3 years or those suspected to have viral tonsillitis.[12]

Please note that neither of these tonsil swabs can differentiate between acute infection and chronic colonization of GAS. Despite adequate treatment, persistent GAS,

Table 2	
Signs and symptoms of viral versus bacterial tonsillitis[10]	
Viral Tonsillitis	**Bacterial Tonsillitis**
Cough	Sudden onset of fever
Rhinorrhea	Sore throat
Conjunctivitis	Dysphagia
	Tonsillar erythema and exudate
	Cervical lymphadenopathy
	Absence of cough
	Strawberry tongue

without active infection or inflammatory response, has been noted for over 1 year. Chronic GAS has little to no risk in developing immune-mediated post-streptococcal complications.[14]

Tonsil swabs
Non-culture-based tests for GAS. A systematic review shows an estimated sensitivity and specificity of 93% and 99% in children versus 95% and 97% in adults for molecular tests. This is compared to immunoassays that show an estimated sensitivity and specificity of 80% and 92% in children versus 91% and 93% in adults.[15] The sensitivity of these tests is dependent on bacterial load and quality of the tonsil swab/throat culture.[12] Serial testing may reduce false negative rates.[12] Due to the almost immediate results, less than 10 minutes, of the non-culture-based tests and its availability at the point of care, these tests aid in timely diagnosis and treatment.[16]

Throat culture. The bacterial culture is the gold standard in the diagnosis of GAS tonsillitis. Although time intensive, often requiring 24 to 72 hours for a result, the sensitivity of the bacterial throat culture is 90% to 95%. These statistics are questionable as they have not been reproduced in clinical practice, only in research laboratories.[3,16]

Other tests to consider
C-reactive protein. Elevated C-reactive protein (CRP) values are most commonly noted in bacterial infections but do not differentiate between upper and lower respiratory tract infections.[17] Elevated CRP 7 days after the onset of symptoms may be more consistent with bacterial infection.[17]

Antistreptolysin O titers. The antistreptolysin O (ASLO) titers are not useful in the diagnosis of acute tonsillitis. It is useful in the diagnosis of ARF, one of the major complications of GAS tonsillitis.[18] Titers should not be ordered to diagnose acute tonsillitis.

Diagnostic imaging. Imaging is rarely indicated for acute, uncomplicated tonsillitis. However, if there are signs of complicated or invasive infection such as unstable vital signs, deviated uvula, drooling, trismus, unilateral facial swelling, or airway compromise, the patient should be redirected to the emergency department for advanced imaging and possible airway management and protection.

TREATMENT

Tonsillitis is usually self-limiting, often caused by viruses rather than bacteria. The mainstay of treatment is supportive care, using acetaminophen and nonsteroidal anti-inflammatory drugs for analgesia. Adequate hydration is also recommended.[19] Patients may return to work or school 24 hours if treatment is indicated.[5]

Acute Tonsillitis

Tonsillitis secondary to bacterial infection will require antibiotic therapy. Group A beta-hemolytic Streptococcus, specifically, requires appropriate and timely treatment to prevent complications. First-line antibiotic choice for GAS tonsillitis is penicillin as noted in **Table 3**. Cephalosporins and macrolides are also effective therapies but only recommended for patients with a true penicillin allergy.[20]

Recurrent Acute Tonsillitis

Recurrent acute tonsillitis, repeated episodes interrupted by intervals without significant symptoms, should be treated with the same antibiotics as noted in **Table 3**. Surgical intervention, tonsillectomy with or without adenoidectomy, is rarely indicated as

Table 3
Antibiotic recommendations for acute and recurrent acute tonsillitis[20,23–26]

Antibiotic	Child Dosage	Adult Dosage	Duration
Penicillin–first line			
Penicillin V	≤ 27 kg 250 mg 2 to 3 times daily >27 kg 500 mg 2 to 3 times daily	500 mg 2 to 3 times daily	10 d
Amoxicillin	50 mg/kg once daily (maximum 1,000 mg dose) Alternative: 25 mg/kg twice daily (maximum 500 mg dose)	250 mg 4 times daily 500 mg twice daily 1,000 mg daily 775 mg extended release once daily	10 d
Penicillin G benzathine	≤ 27 kg 600,000 units intramuscularly >27 kg 1.2 million units intramuscularly	1.2 million units intramuscularly	Once
Cephalosporins			
Cephalexin	40 mg/kg per day divided into twice daily dosage (500 mg maximum dose).	500 mg twice daily	10 d
Cefadroxil	30 mg/kg once daily or divided into twice daily dosage (1000 maximum dose)	1,000 mg daily	10 d
Cefuroxime	10 mg/kg per dose twice daily (250 mg maximum dose)	250 mg twice daily	10 d
Cefpodoxime	5 mg/kg per dose twice daily (100 mg maximum dosage)	100 mg twice daily	5–10 d
Cefdinir	7 mg/kg per dose twice daily 14 mg/kg once daily (600 mg maximum dosage)	300 mg twice daily 600 mg daily	5–10 d for 300 mg 10 days for 600 mg
Macrolides for severe penicillin allergy			
Azithromycin	12 mg/kg per day (500 mg maximum dosage)	12 mg/kg per day (500 mg maximum dosage)	5 d
Clarithromycin	250 mg twice daily	7.5 mg/kg per dose twice daily (250 mg maximum dosage)	10 d

the frequency, severity, and risk of complications of acute tonsillitis decrease with age. The Paradise criteria can guide referral for surgical intervention: 7 or more episodes in 1 year or 5 or more episodes annually over 2 years or 3 or more episodes annually[21,22] over 3 years.[20,23–26]

COMPLEMENTARY AND ALTERNATIVE THERAPIES

Although the Infectious Disease Society of America does not recommend systemic corticosteroids for tonsillitis, the overlap of clinical presentation of viral versus bacterial tonsillitis and other causes of pharyngitis warrant its consideration.[20,27] A single dose of dexamethasone via oral route, 10 mg for adults and 0.6 mg per kg for children with maximum dose of 10 mg, may provide some analgesia and reduce recovery duration for nonspecific pharyngitis.[28]

Drinking hot tea with honey and gargling with salt water have also helped with symptoms of tonsillitis. Honey should not be given to children aged less than 12 months due to the increased risk for botulism. Herbal remedies, homeopathic therapies, and probiotics are neither the Food and Drug Administration regulated nor shown proven efficacy.[29]

COMPLICATIONS
Acute Complications

Acute complications of tonsillitis are due to the extension of the infection into surrounding tissue such as abscess formation. Peritonsillar abscess is a collection of inflammatory concentrate between the pharyngeal constrictor muscle and tonsillar capsule. Patients present with dysphagia, odynophagia, drooling, muffled voice, or trismus. Signs include tonsillar inflammation with uvula deviation away from the affected side.[12] Diagnosis is confirmed with computed tomography (CT) of the head and neck. Definitive treatment should be with incision and drainage, high-dose steroids, and broad-spectrum antibiotics as the etiology tends to be polymicrobial.

Chronic Complications

Without appropriate and timely treatment, tonsillitis can cause lifelong sequelae such as rheumatic fever, post-streptococcal glomerulonephritis (PSGN), and Lemierre syndrome. ARF is an immune-mediated disease that is rarely seen in developed nations. The symptoms of ARF are divided into major and minor criteria, together comprising the Jones criteria. Major criteria include polyarthritis, Sydenham's chorea, clinical and subclinical carditis, erythema marginatum (blanchable, macular rash on trunk, and extremities that is not pruritic), and subcutaneous nodules. Updated Jones criteria include echocardiographic findings to the major criteria.[30] Minor criteria include fever, polyarthralgia, elevated erythrocyte sedimentation rate and CRP, and prolonged PR interval. A positive ASLO or GAS throat swab and 2 major or 1 major with 2 minor Jones criteria are required to diagnose ARF.[31] Supportive care is recommended for patients who do not have signs of carditis and present with only mild arthralgias. Patients who have severe arthralgias or carditis are treated with high-dose aspirin and, in select cases, prednisone with subsequent taper. Antibiotics are only recommended if throat swab is positive. Up to 50% of ARF will result in long-term cardiac sequelae such as mitral valve stenosis.[10]

PSGN may also develop after GAS tonsillitis. It more commonly affects those living in developing nations with higher density communities. Patients present with generalized edema and elevated blood pressure. Signs of renal injury such as proteinuria and electrolyte imbalance may also be present. Since PSGN is an autoimmune disorder, low serum complement levels may also be noted. Fortunately, PSGN is often a self-limiting disease with eventual return to baseline kidney function.[10]

Lemierre syndrome is a rare complication of tonsillitis. It is characterized by septic jugular vein thrombophlebitis or thrombosis secondary to septic emboli. It develops after recurrent tonsillitis secondary to *Fusobacterium necrophorum*, and, less frequently, due to staphylococcal and streptococcal species.[10] It is more common in the pediatric and younger adult populations, presenting with unilateral neck pain with a history of sore throat.[32] Occasionally, patients will also have dysphagia or voice changes. Lemierre syndrome is diagnosed with CT or MRI. Lemierre syndrome is treated with a course of intravenous antibiotics such as ampicillin/sulbactam. Transition from intravenous to oral antibiotics may be considered but it has not been well studied to complete a 6 week course. Anticoagulation is not recommendation and surgery is recommended only if there is further clot development while being treated with antibiotics.[33]

PROGNOSIS

Patients suspected to have viral tonsillitis should expect symptom improvement within 1 to 3 days with supportive therapy. If improvement is not as expected, however, clinicians should reevaluate the patient for bacterial tonsillitis. Although antibiotic therapy has only been shown to reduce symptoms by 16 hours, the appropriate treatment of GAS tonsillitis is required to reduce the development of acute complications and potentially more systemic and serious illness.

CLINICS CARE POINTS

- Acute tonsillitis is a common clinical diagnosis in the pediatric population and accurate speciation is required to drive treatment.
- Modified Centor criteria should be used to ensure appropriate resource utilization and antibiotic stewardship.
- Untreated group A beta-hemolytic Streptococcus tonsillitis can lead to acute rheumatic fever (with up to 50% of cases developing mitral valve stenosis) and post-stroptococcal glomerulonephritis (with usually no long-term sequelae).
- Since tonsillitis is more commonly cuased by viruses, the mainstay of treatment is supportive with analgesics.

DISCLOSURES

The authors have nothing to disclose.

REFERENCES

1. Schappert SM, Rechtsteiner EA. Ambulatory medical care utilization estimates for 2006. Natl Health Stat Report 2008;(8):1–29.
2. Windfuhr JP, Toepfner N, Steffen G, et al. Clinical practice guideline: tonsillitis I. Diagnostics and nonsurgical management. Eur Arch Oto-Rhino-Laryngol 2016; 273:973–87.
3. Mustafa Z, Ghaffari M. Diagnostic methods, clinical guidelines, and antibiotic treatment for group A streptococcal pharyngitis: a narrative review. Front Cell Infect Microbiol 2020;10:563627.

4. Shulman ST, Bisno AL, Clegg HW, et al. Clinical practice guideline for the diagnosis and management of group A streptococcal pharyngitis: 2012 update by the Infectious Diseases Society of America. Clin Infect Dis 2012;55(10):279–82.
5. Ashurst JV and Edgerley-Gibb L. Streptococcal pharyngitis, In: StatPearls [Internet], 2024, StatPearls Publishing; Treasure Island (FL), Available at: https://www.ncbi.nlm.nih.gov/books/NBK525997/ (Accessed 23 October 2024).
6. Scadding GK. Immunology of the tonsil: a review. J R Soc Med 1989;83(2):104–7. https://doi.org/10.1177/014107689008300216.
7. Nave H, Gebert A, Pabst R. Morphology and immunology of the human palatine tonsil. Anat Embryol 2001;204(5):367–73. https://doi.org/10.1007/s004290100210.
8. Putto A. Febrile exudative tonsillitis: viral or streptococcal? Pediatrics 1987; 80:6–12.
9. Smith KL, Hughes R, Myrex P. Tonsillitis and tonsilloliths: diagnosis and management. Am Fam Physician 2023;107(1):35–41.
10. Anderson J, Paterek E. Tonsillitis. StatPearls 2023. Available at: https://www.ncbi.nlm.nih.gov/books/NBK544342/.
11. Cleveland Clinic. Tonsillitis: symptoms, causes & treatment. Cleveland Clinic 2023. Available at: https://my.clevelandclinic.org/health/diseases/21146-tonsillitis. Accessed April 9, 2024.
12. Norton L, Myers A. The treatment of streptococcal tonsillitis/pharyngitis in young children. World journal of otorhinolaryngology - head and neck surgery 2021;7(3): 161–5. Available at: https://www.ncbi.nlm.nih.gov/pmc/articles/PMC8356196/.
13. Willis BH, Coomar D, Baragilly M. Comparison of Centor and McIsaac scores in primary care: a meta-analysis over multiple thresholds. Br J Gen Pract 2020; 70(693):e245–54 [Erratum appears in Br J Gen Pract 2020;70(694):230]. PMID: 32152041; PMCID: PMC7065683.
14. Tanz RR, Shulman ST. Chronic pharyngeal carriage of group A streptococci. Pediatr Infect Dis J 2007;26(2):175–6.
15. Banerjee S, Ford C. Rapid tests for the diagnosis of group a streptococcal infection: a review of diagnostic test accuracy, clinical utility, safety, and cost-effectiveness [Internet]. Ottawa (Ontario): Canadian Agency for Drugs and Technologies in Health; 2018. Available at: https://www.ncbi.nlm.nih.gov/books/NBK532707/.
16. Rao A, Berg B, Quezada T, et al. Diagnosis and antibiotic treatment of group a streptococcal pharyngitis in children in a primary care setting: impact of point-of-care polymerase chain reaction. BMC Pediatr 2019;19(1):24. PMID: 30651115; PMCID: PMC6335697.
17. Melbye H, Hvidsten D, Holm A, et al. The course of C-reactive protein response in untreated upper respiratory tract infection. Br J Gen Pract 2004;54(506):653–8. PMID: 15353049; PMCID: PMC1326064.
18. Geerts I, De Vos N, Frans J, et al. The clinical-diagnostic role of antistreptolysin o antibodies. Acta Clin Belg 2011;66(6):410–5.
19. Stelter K. Tonsillitis and sore throat in children. GMS Curr Top Otorhinolaryngol, Head Neck Surg 2014;13:Doc07. Available at: https://www.ncbi.nlm.nih.gov/pmc/articles/PMC4273168/.
20. Shulman ST, Bisno AL, Clegg HW, et al. Clinical practice guideline for the diagnosis and management of group A streptococcal pharyngitis: 2012 update by the Infectious Diseases Society of America. Clin Infect Dis 2012;55(10):1279–82 [Published correction appears in Clin Infect Dis 2014;58(10):1496].
21. Mitchell RB, Archer SM, Ishman SL, et al. Clinical practice guideline: tonsillectomy in children (update). Otolaryngol Head Neck Surg 2019;160(1_suppl):S1–42.

22. Paradise JL, Bluestone CD, Bachman RZ, et al. Efficacy of tonsillectomy for recurrent throat infection in severely affected children. Results of parallel randomized and nonrandomized clinical trials. N Engl J Med 1984;310(11):674–83. PMID: 6700642.
23. Van Driel ML, De Sutter AI, Thorning S, et al. Different antibiotic treatments for group A streptococcal pharyngitis. Cochrane Database Syst Rev 2021;(3): CD004406.
24. Spinks A, Glasziou PP, Del Mar CB. Antibiotics for sore throat. Cochrane Database Syst Rev 2013;(11):CD000023.
25. Lexicomp. Available at: https://online.lexi.com/lco/action/login. Accessed June 16, 2022.
26. National Institute for Health and Care Excellence. Sore throat (acute): antimicrobial prescribing. 2018. Available at: https://www.nice.org.uk/guidance/ng84. Accessed June 15, 2021.
27. Aertgeerts B, Agoritsas T, Siemieniuk RAC, et al. Corticosteroids for sore throat: a clinical practice guideline. BMJ 2017;358:j4090.
28. Sadeghirad B, Siemieniuk RAC, Brignardello-Petersen R, et al. Corticosteroids for treatment of sore throat: systematic review and meta-analysis of randomised trials. BMJ 2017;358:j3887.
29. Bereznoy VV, Riley DS, Wassmer G, et al. Efficacy of extract of Pelargonium sidoides in children with acute non-group A beta-hemolytic streptococcus tonsillopharyngitis: a randomized, double-blind, placebo-controlled trial. Alternative Ther Health Med 2003;9(5):68–79. PMID: 14526713.
30. Gewitz MH, Baltimore RS, Tani LY, et al. Revision of the Jones Criteria for the diagnosis of acute rheumatic fever in the era of Doppler echocardiography: a scientific statement from the American Heart Association. Circulation 2015;131(20): 1806–18. PMID: 25908771.
31. Majmundar VD and Nagalli S. Erythema marginatum, In: *StatPearls [Internet]*, 2024, StatPearls Publishing; Treasure Island (FL), Available at: https://www.ncbi.nlm.nih.gov/books/NBK557835/ (Accessed 23 October 2024).
32. Holm K, Bank S, Nielsen H, et al. The role of Fusobacterium necrophorum in pharyngotonsillitis – a review. Anaerobe 2016;42:89–97. PMID:27693542.
33. Bondy P, Grant T. Lemierre's syndrome: what are the roles for anticoagulation and long-term antibiotic therapy? Ann Otol Rhinol Laryngol 2008;117(9):679–83. PMID:18834071.

Rhinitis in Primary Care

Nirali Patel, DO, MS[a,b,*], Adity Bhattacharyya, MD[b,c]

KEYWORDS

- Rhinitis • Allergic rhinitis • Subtypes • Diagnosis • Treatment

KEY POINTS

- Rhinitis is a prevalent ailment affecting millions of people across the world with allergic rhinitis being the most common etiology.
- The diagnosis is mostly clinical, though testing may be needed to identify the causative agent.
- Topical agents like intranasal corticosteroids or inhaled antihistamines are the first-line therapies for both allergic and nonallergic rhinitis.
- Persistent symptoms of rhinitis can be targeted with specific therapy to provide relief.

INTRODUCTION

Rhinitis is defined as the presence of one of the following symptoms: rhinorrhea, nasal stuffiness, nasal itching, sneezing, or cough. It is extremely common and affects everyone some time in their life. Rhinitis may be present on its own or be a part of other disease syndromes.[1]

Epidemiology

Rhinitis is very prevalent, and the rates of allergic rhinitis (AR) are 10% to 30% of adults and 40% of children in the United States with some estimates suggesting up to 400 million people worldwide are affected.[1,2] The rates are much higher in patients who suffer from asthma. AR is present in 75% of patients with asthma and is present in almost all patients with the diagnosis of allergic asthma. It affects the quality of life in most patients, and symptoms caused by rhinitis include disturbed sleep, daytime sleepiness, impaired attention, irritability as well as learning and memory deficits. This causes significant loss of work and school days as well a loss of productivity, especially on days when allergies are at their worst levels.[3]

According to the Global Asthma Network Phase I, the overall prevalence of rhinoconjunctivitis is 13.3% in adolescents and 7.7% in children studied across 25

[a] Family Medicine Department, JFK University Medical Center, 65 James Street, Edison, NJ 08820, USA; [b] Family Medicine Residency Program, Edison, NJ, USA; [c] Family Medicine Department, JFK University Medical Center
* Corresponding author. Family Medicine Department, JFK University Medical Center, 65 James Street, Edison, NJ 08820.
E-mail address: niralim.patel@hmhn.org

Prim Care Clin Office Pract 52 (2025) 37–45
https://doi.org/10.1016/j.pop.2024.09.006
0095-4543/25/© 2024 Elsevier Inc. All rights reserved, including those for text and data mining, AI training, and similar technologies.

countries.[4,5] Of note, there was high variability noted among the different countries. Environmental factors such as pollution, mold, window condensation, incense use, and other factors were associated with the higher prevalence, in a study conducted in China with a $P<.05$.[6]

Cost of Health Care

It is difficult to ascertain the actual cost to treat a patient with AR. There are estimates that up to 70% of individuals may purchase over-the-counter medications to treat their symptoms with or without an official diagnosis.[7,8] Productivity losses were calculated by Crystal-Peters and colleagues, using data from the National Health Interviews Study (NHIS) including the use of sedating over-the-counter allergy medications and worker's self-assessment regarding productivity.[9] The cost was estimated to be up to $5.2 billion per year, and this was partly due to survey participants reporting the sedative effects of the medications as a contributing factor.[9–11]

Types of Rhinitis

There are multiple types of rhinitis but the common ones are as follows.

1. Allergic rhinitis
2. Nonallergic rhinitis (NAR)
3. Rhinitis of pregnancy
4. Occupational rhinitis
5. Atrophic rhinitis

Allergic Rhinitis

This is the commonest type of rhinitis and can be intermittent AR, seasonal AR (SAR), or perennial AR (PAR) depending on the offending agent. Most patients complain of nasal congestion, watery nasal discharge, itching, and sneezing. Nasal itching differentiates AR from other types. Patients may complain of fatigue and poor sleep. Many also complain of snoring and frequent headaches.[1,3]

Examination of the nasal mucosa may be pale and edematous but may also be normal. Children may have purplish discoloration under the eyes called *allergic shiners* and a nasal crease on top of the nose from constant rubbing due to nasal itching.[3]

Nonallergic Rhinitis

NAR is often a diagnosis of exclusion and presents with nasal stuffiness, rhinorrhea, and postnasal drip. Itching of the eyes and nose are notably absent. Typical triggers for NAR are strong odors like cigarette smoke, perfumes, exhaust fumes from cars, and cleaning products.[1] Children with NAR tend to have milder nasal symptoms with a less severe clinical course.[4] Special types of NAR are: *vasomotor rhinitis (VMR)* which is rhinorrhea in response to cold dry air or temperature changes and *gustatory rhinitis* which is rhinorrhea in response to eating spicy foods caused by vagal responses.

Rhinitis medicamentosa

This condition is caused by overuse of over-the-counter nasal decongestant sprays, such as oxymetazoline and xylometazoline, that cause rebound congestion after stopping. However, its presentation and development are inconsistent where it may occur within 3 days of use or may not develop after 6 weeks of use.[1] This leads to a vicious cycle of overuse and dependency on these nasal sprays. On a physical examination, the nasal mucosa is swollen red and inflamed.[4]

Medication-induced rhinitis

Many commonly used medications can cause rhinitis, making it important to take a good medication history when patients complain of chronic rhinorrhea. These include antihypertensive medications like the alpha-blocker clonidine, angiotensin-converting enzyme inhibitors, calcium channel blockers, and thiazide diuretics. Medications used for erectile dysfunction, antidepressants, benzodiazepines, psychotropic medications, and certain antiseizure medications like gabapentin can also cause rhinorrhea.[1]

Rhinitis of Pregnancy

This is a diagnosis of exclusion. Rhinitis occurs in the last 2 months of pregnancy when all other causes are excluded and the condition resolves after 2 weeks of delivery, which is classified as rhinitis of pregnancy.[12,13] The exact mechanism in pregnancy is unknown but may be due to an increase in estrogen and progesterone. Estrogen can lead to nasal vascular engorgement causing congestion, and both estrogen and progesterone can increase eosinophil migration.[1]

Occupational Rhinitis

Occupational rhinitis is caused by exposure to irritants or allergens that are specific to a patient's place of work. Patients complain of resolution of symptoms when they are away from work, like on weekends.[1]

Alcohol-induced rhinitis

Some people complain of rhinorrhea after alcohol ingestion. This is seen in some healthy individuals but is much more common in asthmatics and patients with aspirin allergies. It is an exaggerated response of alcohol-induced vasodilation and is more common with individuals who drink wine.[1]

Atrophic Rhinitis

This typically occurs in the elderly who have had repeated nasal or sinus procedures. The nasal mucosa is atrophic and gets colonized with bacteria which causes a bad odor and crusting besides nasal congestion with a dry feeling.[13]

Recreational drug use

The use of intranasal recreational drugs like heroin and cocaine can also cause chronic rhinorrhea and should be included in the broad differential diagnosis. No clear studies indicate the quantity and duration of recreational drug use that may lead to the development of rhinitis.

Systemic diseases

Many systemic diseases may have presentations that include rhinorrhea. Most of these diseases involve the sinuses as well and are not limited to the nose. Some of these diseases include hypothyroidism, cystic fibrosis, granulomatous polyangiitis, and sarcoidosis.[1]

DIAGNOSIS

Rhinitis is considered a clinical diagnosis. For AR, there is no gold standard and little definitive diagnostic criteria.[2] Consensus states that initial diagnosis can be made if there is a known allergen exposure with greater than or equal to 2 of the following symptoms: nasal congestion, nasal pruritus, rhinorrhea, or sneezing. Experts recommend an immunoglobulin E (IgE)-mediated hypersensitivity skin testing (aeroallergen skin prick test) to confirm the diagnosis and offending agent, if there is a strong history consistent with AR. If greater than or equal to 2 symptoms persist for greater than or equal to 1 hour per day for greater than or equal to 12 weeks, then it is categorized as chronic rhinosinusitis (CRS).[14]

In all patients, clinical history should be obtained, which includes questions regarding symptom severity, duration, and frequency. Patient-specific questions are important such as age of onset, pattern of presentation, triggers (or suspected triggers), timing during the year, and progression of each individual symptom. Family history and personal medical history should include asthma and other rhinitis-associated conditions, or conditions that mimic rhinitis such as nasal septal wall abnormalities, turbinate hypertrophy, adenoidal hypertrophy, nasal tumors, nasal polyps (with or without chronic rhinitis), nasal collapse, primary ciliary dyskinesia, and pharyngeal reflux.[1]

Physical examination with appropriate equipment (nasal speculum, otoscopy with nasal adaptor) can be used to narrow down the differentials. In patients with chronic rhinitis without atopy or positive allergy testing, it may indicate NAR. Further differentiation of subtypes can be done via nasal provocation test with allergen, microbiologic and cytologic evaluation, and assessing IgE levels in the nasal cavity.[1,4,14–16] If there are suspected structural or functional abnormalities, the lack of improvement with treatment, or other complications, patients should be referred to ENT or allergist for further testing.

Some experts' statements suggest using validated questionnaires to assess the severity of patients' symptomatology to help guide treatment; however, the certainty of evidence is low. There are several validated questionnaires including the Sinonasal Outcome Test (SNOT-22) which focuses on quality of life and symptom control for patients with AR.[17] The Visual Analog Scale can be utilized to assess the severity of rhinitis which are in line with the "Allergic Rhinitis and its Impact on Asthma" (ARIA) guidelines.[18]

TREATMENT
Allergic Rhinitis

When possible, avoiding allergen exposure and triggering factors is the first step. Per the ARIA initiative guidelines and expert opinion, first-line therapy is oral or intranasal antihistamine (INAH), such as azelastine, for mild AR and SAR.[1,19] Second-generation oral antihistamines are generally preferred over first-generation antihistamines to avoid potential side effects of sedation, poor sleep quality, and more specifically anticholinergic side effects.[1] Patients can utilize intranasal cromolyn prior to being exposed to triggering allergies to mitigate the subsequent rhinitis symptoms.[1,15,16]

In the case of persistent AR, moderate AR, or severe AR, intranasal corticosteroid is the first-line and preferred monotherapy. Some experts recommend using a combination of intranasal corticosteroid (INCS) and INAH for moderate and severe SAR symptoms.[1,4,14–16]

There is low evidence on the efficacy of oral leukotriene receptor antagonists (LTRA), such as montelukast or zafilukast, and expert opinion does not recommend its use for the initial treatment of AR unless the patient cannot tolerate alternative therapies.[1] Studies have shown, however, that LTRAs are effective in treating chronic SAR and PAR. Expert opinion recommends its use for patients who suffer from both AR and asthma.[1] Oral corticosteroid therapy can be used in very severe AR or in cases that are not improving, but the evidence is poor.[1]

Depending on specific symptoms, additional therapies can be utilized. Intranasal ipratropium has been noted to help with rhinorrhea in conjunction with INCS.

Intranasal decongestants can be used for short-term treatment for severe mucosal edema which may be preventing other medications from being effective. Of note, it is not routinely used due to side effects such as rhinitis medicamentosa. Comparatively, oral decongestant may help to relieve nasal congestion without causing dependence. For asthmatic patients suffering from AR, the combination of oral decongestant and second-generation oral antihistamines may significantly help relieve symptoms.[1]

Nasal irrigation with saline can be utilized to moisten dry nasal passages, reduce inflammation, increase mucociliary clearance, and clear mucosal passages of blood and mucus. However, contamination in the devices used can lead to worsening CRS via backwash or lead to exposure of bacteria or parasites if contaminated tap water is being used. It is, therefore, important that patients carefully follow the instructions written on the saline irrigation bottles to avoid contamination.[1,7,20]

First-line therapy for CRS is topical nasal saline and topical nasal corticosteroid spray. Hypertonic saline (nasal saline irrigation) was found to be more effective over isotonic solution in CRS.[7,20] Of note, if individuals have nasal polyps then intranasal corticosteroids are considered the first-line treatment.[21]

Patients with moderate or severe AR can be referred for allergen immunotherapy (AIT) if symptoms are not well controlled with initial measures of avoiding allergens or other pharmacotherapy. Additionally, immunotherapy may reduce the severity of other comorbid conditions such as asthma.[1]

Nonallergic Rhinitis

First-line therapy is INCS or INAH. First- and second-generation antihistamines can be used in VMR and NAR to treat nasal congestion, postnasal drainage, and rhinorrhea. Inhaled ipratropium has been found to be effective in decreasing symptoms of rhinorrhea, but LTRA are not effective. In moderate and severe NAR that is resistant to monotherapy, the combination of INCS and INAH can be very effective.[1,13,22]

SPECIAL POPULATIONS

For pediatric patients, treatment is focused on avoiding triggers/allergens, immunotherapy, and pharmacotherapy. Therapy regimen is like the adults as written earlier. Patients as young as 2 years old can be treated with fluticasone INCS, loratadine oral antihistamine, and intranasal cromolyn. There is a low likelihood that patients under the age of 2 years old exhibit signs of AR. Intranasal histamines and some sublingual immunotherapies are available for children greater than 5 years old.

In pregnant patients, nasal saline is considered first-line therapy. As of 2015, the FDA replaced the previously used pregnancy category classification (A, B, C, X) allowing for more discussion regarding safety and use. Many medications used to treat rhinitis fall under the B and C categories. "Category B" designate animal studies have shown no risk to the fetus, but there are no adequate studies in humans, and "Category C" show an adverse effect to the fetus, but no adequate studies in humans are available—but the benefits may out weight the risks. Most INCS are well tolerated, except for triamcinolone (INCS) which is contraindicated (category C). Oral second-generation antihistamines (such as diphenhydramine, cetirizine, and loratadine—category B), INAHs (limited data), intranasal cromolyn (category B), LTRA (such as montelukast—category B), and intranasal ipratropium (category B) are considered low risk in pregnancy in limited studies. Oral decongestants should be avoided during the first trimester of pregnancy and cautiously used in the second and third trimesters.[1,23,24]

Table 1
Common medication treatments in rhinitis

Therapy Type	Mechanism of Action	Condition Treated	Comments
First-generation antihistamine	Nonselectively antagonize central and peripheral histamine H1 receptors	NAR	NAR
Second-generation antihistamine	Selectively antagonize peripheral H1 receptors	All subtypes of allergic rhinitis	First-line for mild allergic rhinitis Recommended over first-generation antihistamines
Intranasal antihistamine (INAH)	Antagonizes central and peripheral H1 receptors (nonselective antihistamine)	Intermittent rhinitis, seasonal allergic rhinitis, nonallergic rhinitis	First line for mild allergic rhinitis
Oral steroid	Inhibits multiple inflammatory cytokines	Intractable or very severe allergic rhinitis	Short-term course (5–7 d) only
Intranasal corticosteroid (INCS)	Inhibits multiple inflammatory cytokines	Persistent allergic rhinitis	First line for persistent allergic rhinitis, chronic rhinitis, and NAR
Intranasal decongestants	Stimulates smooth muscle alpha-adrenergic receptors, causing vasoconstriction	Severe mucosal edema	By decreasing mucosal edema other medications can then be delivered Short-term therapy only
Oral decongestants	Stimulates smooth muscle alpha-adrenergic receptors, causing vasoconstriction	Allergic rhinitis	Helps relieve nasal congestion High side effect profile in older adults and children <4 years old. Avoid in pregnancy.
Intranasal ipratropium	Antagonizes acetyl-choline receptors, inhibiting nasal serous/seromucous gland secretions	Perennial and chronic AR and NAR	Effective for reducing rhinorrhea
Intranasal cromolyn	Inhibits mass cell degranulation	Allergic rhinitis	Recommended to use prior to exposure to allergen
Leukotriene receptor antagonist	Selectively binds to cysteinyl leukotriene receptors, decreasing inflammation and swelling	Allergic rhinitis, patients with comorbid asthma	Not recommended for initial treatment of allergic rhinitis Useful in patients with comorbid allergic rhinitis and asthma
Combination of INCS and INAH	Inhibits multiple inflammatory cytokines; antagonizes central and peripheral H1 receptors	Moderate and severe allergic rhinitis, NAR	Effective in patients who are resistant to monotherapy
Combination of INCS with intranasal ipratropium	Suppression of polymorphonuclear leukocyte migraine and reversing increased permeability	Persistent rhinorrhea	Effective for persistent rhinorrhea
Nasal saline	Moisturize nasal passages and clear mucus	All rhinitis subtypes	Can be used in all ages. Preferred therapy for pregnant patients due to relatively low side effect profile
Allergen immunotherapy	Improve tolerance to allergen via exposure therapy	Moderate or severe allergic rhinitis	Can be useful therapy for patients whose symptoms are not well controlled on other therapy.

Information is derived from expert opinion and studies.[1]
Abbreviations: AR, allergic rhinitis; NAR, nonallergic rhinitis.

COMPLEMENTARY AND ALTERNATIVE TREATMENT

There is a growing population of patients interested in nonpharmacologic options for the treatment. Evidence remains inconsistent with limited accurate and reliable data. However, clinicians may offer acupuncture for some patients, taking into account that many cultures incorporate a level of these practices as noted in the Clinical Practice Guidelines Otolaryngology, and Head and Neck Surgery.[10,25] The World Health Organization estimated that up to 80% of the global population may utilize some aspects of complementary and alternative treatment.[25–28] Targeted acupuncture of the sphenopalatine ganglion acupoint may be helpful.[25–28] Another modality of treatment recommended is the use of osteopathic manipulative treatment. Techniques recommended include lymphatic pump techniques, rib raising, thoracic inlet and outlet release, with the goal of correcting cervical dysfunction that may be preventing lymphatic drainage and increased muscle tone causing associated congestion and headaches.[29,30] Future studies and more evidence is needed to address the effectiveness of these specific treatment modalities, but some of them may be beneficial.[29,31]

See **Table 1** for a summary of recommendations.

SUMMARY

Rhinitis is a prevalent symptom and affects most people, sometime during their life. AR is the most common type, especially in patients who also have asthma. It is an expensive burden on the health care system, both in terms of financial costs of treatment and missed days at work. The diagnosis in most cases is clinical and a good history and physical examination is the key to identifying causative agents. The treatment is geared toward avoiding the offending agent and treating the resulting mucosal inflammation. Topical agents like intranasal corticosteroids and inhaled antihistamines are the first-line therapies. If these are not effective, the addition of oral antihistamines is the next step. The second-generation H1 blockers are preferred due to their favorable side effect profile. Leukotriene inhibitors are the third-line agents and are used in patients with AR, especially those with history of asthma.

Patients with moderate to severe symptoms that are persistent can be referred to allergists for AIT. There is little evidence to support the role of oral steroids for the treatment of AR.

CLINICS CARE POINTS

- Rhinitis is mostly a clinical diagnosis, and a good, detailed history is usually sufficient to identify causes and plan appropriate testing.

- Referral to an allergist or otorhinolaryngologist is recommended if symptoms persist despite adequate initial management or further testing is required.

- Topical agents like intranasal corticosteroids or inhaled antihistamines are the first-line therapies for both allergic and nonallergic rhinitis.

- Treatment is stepwise, with the addition of oral second-generation antihistamines and intranasal ipratropium if initial treatment is not adequate.

- There is low evidence on the efficacy of oral leukotriene receptor antagonists and should only be used for the treatment of allergic rhinitis unless the patient cannot tolerate alternative therapies.

- There is a very little evidence for the use of oral corticosteroids in the treatment cf rhinitis and should be avoided.

DISCLOSURE

The authors have nothing to disclose.

REFERENCES

1. Dykewicz MS, Wallace DV, Amrol DJ, et al. Rhinitis 2020: a practice parameter update. J Allergy Clin Immunol 2020;146:721.
2. Nur Husna SM, Tan HT, Md Shukri N, et al. Allergic rhinitis: a clinical and patho-physiological overview. Front Med 2022;9:874114.
3. Meltzer EO, Nathan R, Derebery J, et al. Sleep, quality of life, and productivity impact of nasal symptoms in the United States: findings from the Burden of Rhinitis in America survey. Allergy Asthma Proc 2009;30(3):244–54.
4. Yum HY, Ha EK, Shin YH, et al. Prevalence, comorbidities, diagnosis, and treatment of nonallergic rhinitis: real-world comparison with allergic rhinitis. Clin Exp Pediatr 2021;64(8):373–83.
5. Romero-Tapia S, Garcia-Marcos L. Global burden of pediatric asthma and rhinitis - what we have recently learned from epidemiology. Curr Opin Allergy Clin Immunol 2024;24(3):177–81.
6. Li S, Wu W, Wang G, et al. Association between exposure to air pollution and risk of allergic rhinitis: a systematic review and meta-analysis. Environ Res 2022;205: 112472.
7. Dierick BJH, van der Molen T, Flokstra-de Blok BMJ, et al. Burden and socioeconomics of asthma, allergic rhinitis, atopic dermatitis and food allergy. Expert Rev Pharmacoecon Outcomes Res 2020;20(5):437–53.
8. Tan R, Cvetkovski B, Kritikos V, et al. Identifying the hidden burden of allergic rhinitis (AR) in community pharmacy: a global phenomenon. Asthma Res Pract 2017;3:8.
9. Crystal-Peters J, Crown WH, Goetzel RZ, et al. The cost of productiv ty losses associated with allergic rhinitis. Am J Manag Care 2000;6(3):373–8.
10. Seidman MD, Gurgel RK, Lin SY, et al. Clinical practice guideline: allergic rhinitis. Otolaryngol Head Neck Surg 2015;152(S1):S1–43.
11. Blaiss MS. Allergic rhinitis: direct and indirect costs. Allergy Asthma Proc 2010; 31:375–80.
12. Vaidyanathan S, Williamson P, Clearie K, et al. Fluticasone reverses oxymetazoline-induced tachyphylaxis of response and rebound congestion. Am J Respir Crit Care Med 2010;182(1):19–24.
13. Liva GA, Karatzanis AD, Prokopakis EP. Review of rhinitis: classification, types, pathophysiology. J Clin Med 2021;10(14):3183.
14. Testera-Montes A, Jurado R, Salas M, et al. Diagnostic tools in allergic rhinitis. Front Allergy 2021;2:721851.
15. Schultz A, Stuck B, Feuring M, et al. Novel approaches in the treatment of allergic rhinitis. Curr Opin Allergy Clin Immunol 2003;3(1):21–7.
16. Eguiluz-Gracia I, Pérez-Sánchez N, Bogas G, et al. How to diagnose and treat local allergic rhinitis: a challenge for clinicians. J Clin Med 2019;8(7):1062.
17. Husain Q, Hoehle L, Phillips K, et al. The 22-item sinonasal Outcome tes: as a tool for the assessment of quality of life and symptom control in allergic rhinitis. Am J Rhinol Allergy 2020;34(2):209–16.

18. Bousquet PJ, Combescure C, Neukirch F, et al. Visual analog scales can assess the severity of rhinitis graded according to ARIA guidelines. Allergy 2007;62(4): 367–72.
19. Klimek L, Bachert C, Pfaar O, et al. ARIA guideline 2019: treatment of allergic rhinitis in the German health system. Allergol Select 2019;3(1):22–50.
20. Huang A, Govindaraj S. Topical therapy in the management of chronic rhinosinusitis. Curr Opin Otolaryngol Head Neck Surg 2013;21(1):31–8.
21. Fokkens W, Lund V, Mullol J. European Position Paper on Rhinosinusitis and Nasal Polyps Group, EP³OS 2007: European position paper on rhinosinusitis and nasal polyps 2007: a summary for otorhinolaryngologists. Rhinology 2007; 45:97–101.
22. Hellings PW, Klimek L, Cingi C, et al. Non-allergic rhinitis: position paper of the European academy of allergy and clinical immunology. Allergy 2017;72(11): 1657–65.
23. Ellegård EK. Pregnancy rhinitis. Immunol Allergy Clin North Am 2006;26(1): 119–135,vii.
24. Weaver-Agostoni J, Kosak Z and Bartlett S. Allergic rhinitis: rapid evidence review. AAFP, Available at: https://www.aafp.org/pubs/afp/issues/2023/0500/allergic-rhinitis.html (Accessed 15 May 2024).
25. Guo Y, Cai S, Deng J, et al. Trends and hotspots of acupuncture for allergic rhinitis: a bibliometric analysis from 2002 to 2022. Compl Ther Med 2023;78: 102984.
26. Fu Q, Zhang L, Liu Y, et al. Effectiveness of acupuncturing at the sphenopalatine ganglion acupoint alone for treatment of allergic rhinitis: a systematic review and meta-analysis. Evid base Compl Alternative Med 2019;2019:6478102.
27. Witt CM, Brinkhaus B. Efficacy, effectiveness and cost-effectiveness of acupuncture for allergic rhinitis – an overview about previous and ongoing studies. Auton Neurosci 2010;157(1–2):42–5.
28. World Health Organization, WHO traditional medicine strategy: 2014-2023, Available at: http://www.who.int/iris/bitstream/10665/92455/1/9789241506090_eng.pdf?ua=1.A (Accessed 15 May 2024).
29. Wu S, Graven K, Sergi M, et al. Rhinitis: the osteopathic modular approach. J Osteopath Med 2020;120(5):351–8.
30. Bukhari O, Phillips G, Sweeney K. Non-allergic rhinitis with osteopathic treatment techniques. Osteopathic Family Physician 2020;12(2):16–20.
31. Bielory L. Complementary and alternative medicine in allergy-immunology: more information is needed. J Allergy Clin Immunol Pract 2018;6(1):99–100.

Obstructive Sleep Apnea

Nicholas Anderson, MD[a],*, Patty Tran, DO[b]

KEYWORDS

- Obstructive sleep apnea • Adult • Pediatric • Diagnosis • Treatment

KEY POINTS

- Obstructive sleep apnea (OSA) is a commonly underdiagnosed heterogenous condition that causes a significant burden of disease across the world.
- OSA causes significant long-term sequelae beyond just significant daytime sleepiness.
- Recognition of OSA and implementation of appropriate testing and treatment at the primary care level is crucial.
- Diagnostic methods for OSA, particularly at home testing options, are rapidly changing and becoming more convenient for patients.
- While positive airway pressure (PAP) therapy remains the mainstay of treatment for OSA, other exciting viable treatment options have emerged for those who cannot tolerate PAP therapy.

HISTORY

It is a common belief that sleep apnea syndrome was first described by Charles Dickens in his novel "The Pickwick Papers" (1836), which featured a character who exhibited obesity, loud snoring, and somnolence.[1] However, there were references to sleep disturbances dated back as far as 400 BC when Hippocrates noted the consequences of disrupted sleep on long-term health.[2] Until the late nineteenth century, research on sleep apnea symptoms focused solely on patients' obesity rather than the disordered breathing they experienced during sleep.

In 1965, the first polysomnography (PSG) was used by French researchers Gastaut, Tassinari, and Duron to observe apneic events during sleep, marking a crucial advancement in sleep apnea research. In 1970, the first sleep clinic was established by William Dement at Stanford University in California. Two years later, Christian Guilleminault joined the clinic and his research focused on respiratory disorders during sleep. Ever since, there has been an intense growth of sleep apnea research,

[a] Sleep and Insomnia Center, Hawaii Pacific Neuroscience, Honolulu, HI, USA; [b] Department of Family Medicine and Community Health (DFMCH), John A Burns School of Medicine, University of Hawaii, 98-1005 Moanalua Road, Suite 3030, Aiea, HI 96701, USA
* Corresponding author. 2230 Liliha St #104, Honolulu, HI 96817.
E-mail address: nanderson@hawaiineuroscience.com

Prim Care Clin Office Pract 52 (2025) 47–59
https://doi.org/10.1016/j.pop.2024.09.007 **primarycare.theclinics.com**
0095-4543/25/© 2024 Elsevier Inc. All rights reserved, including those for text and data mining, AI training, and similar technologies.

especially during 1975 to 1980, with more than 300 articles on sleep apnea published in the literature.[3]

In 1980, Dr Colin Sullivan from Sydney, Australia, who devoted his career to studying respiratory control in dogs, invented the first continuous positive airway pressure (CPAP) machine, revolutionizing the treatment of sleep apnea. The treatment was not widely accepted by the public in the beginning. It was not until almost 20 years later, in 2000, when 4 separate papers were published in the same year that found significant sleep apnea-related health effects, a turning point in sleep apnea studies occurred. Later studies also showed a strong association between sleep apnea and an increased prevalence of a range of comorbidities such as hypertension, coronary heart disease, heart failure, and stroke.[3]

EPIDEMIOLOGY

Obstructive sleep apnea (OSA) is highly underdiagnosed in the United States, with 82% of men and 93% of women with OSA unaware of their conditions.[4] Estimates of prevalence vary depending on diagnostic methods, definitions of the disease, age, gender, body mass index (BMI), and racial backgrounds.[5]

The prevalence of OSA increases with age and appears to plateau in the elderly group. Men are twice as likely to develop OSA, although this difference declines in the middle to older age group, as menopause is a risk factor for OSA. Compared with Whites, the prevalence of OSA is higher in Blacks and similar in Asians. Despite generally having a lower BMI, differences in craniofacial bony structures predispose Asians to developing OSA. Although there is limited data on OSA prevalence rates among Hispanic and Native Americans, there is evidence that OSA prevalence has increased in these groups, likely due to rising obesity rates.[5]

In the pediatric population, the prevalence is estimated between 1% and 4%, although this is likely underestimated given the obesity epidemic. There is no gender difference in prevalence for prepubertal children, but it is more prevalent in adolescent males compared with females. OSA is more prevalent in Black children compared with White children, but the prevalence among other ethnicities has not been well established to this point.

PATHOPHYSIOLOGY

The 2 most common types of sleep apneas are obstructive and central sleep apnea. Central sleep apnea (CSA) results from dysfunction in the respiratory control centers of the brainstem, which fail to provide signals to inhale, causing the individual to miss one or more breathing cycles during sleep. In contrast, OSA occurs when there is a physical blockage of the upper airway despite the brain sending signals to breathe.[6]

The pathophysiology of OSA is complex but the underlying etiology involves the upper airway dilating muscles becoming insufficient to prevent narrowing and/or closure of the upper airway during sleep. During inspiration, the negative pressure generated in the lumen of the upper airway promotes closure, and pharyngeal dilating muscles must counteract this force to maintain airway patency.[7] Conditions that elevate negative pressure within the upper airway or impair the ability of dilating muscles to maintain airway patency disrupt this equilibrium, increasing the likelihood of upper airway obstruction.[8]

Upper Airway Narrowing

The most prominent factors contributing to upper airway narrowing are either excessive bulk of soft tissue (tongue, soft palate, and lateral pharyngeal walls) from obesity or craniofacial anatomy, or both.[7] Adenotonsillar hypertrophy, often linked to obesity, is a major risk factor for pediatric OSA.[8]

Volume overload from congestive heart failure (CHF) or end-stage renal disease (ESRD) results in fluid redistribution to the parapharyngeal soft tissues in the recumbent position, which can increase upper airway resistance and collapsibility.[8]

Additional factors, such as nasal obstruction (as seen in rhinitis), the use of intranasal corticosteroids, and the supine posture, have also been identified as adverse influences on upper airway patency.[8]

In pediatric populations, the primary cause of airway narrowing is due to adenotonsillar hypertrophy, although abnormal neuromuscular control also contributes to the development of OSA, like adults.

Upper Airway Dilator Muscle Function

In rapid eye movement (REM) sleep, especially during phasic REM, there is an additional decrease in tone and phasic activity of the pharyngeal dilating muscle, which likely exacerbates the length and severity of apneas and hypopneas.[7]

Apnea Threshold

The apnea threshold is the partial pressure of carbon dioxide ($Paco_2$) at which respiratory effort ceases and apnea occurs and reflects the system's sensitivity to changes in carbon dioxide levels. Patients with OSA and a low apneic threshold have an increased likelihood of apneic events during sleep, as minor fluctuations in $Paco_2$ can trigger airway collapse or respiratory instability.[9]

Loop-Gain

Loop-gain refers to the ratio of the ventilatory response to the disturbance causing it and is a reflection of the sensitivity and responsiveness to changes in ventilation. In patients with OSA, a high loop-gain results in an exaggerated response to respiratory disturbances, which in turn causes unstable ventilation and oscillations in breathing resulting in recurrent hypoxia.[10,11]

Apnea Resolution

Apneas/hypopneas resolve due to 2 mechanisms: The first is increased upper airway muscle tone secondary to chemical (low Pao_2, high $Paco_2$) or mechanical stimuli (stretching of mechanoreceptors). The second mechanism is an arousal from sleep which causes a shift out of the sleep state, thus restoring muscle activity seen during the wake state.

Disease Course

Long-term population studies have shown that OSA severity gradually progresses over time.[7] Weight gain over time similarly results in worsened OSA severity. Conversely, weight loss results in decreased OSA severity. However, weight gain has a greater impact on OSA severity than weight loss, and weight impacts are greater in men compared with women.[7]

Long-term Complications of Obstructive Sleep Apnea

OSA has been identified as a significant risk factor in cardiovascular disease including essential hypertension, coronary artery disease, CHF, pulmonary hypertension, stroke, cardiac arrhythmias, and premature mortality.[7,12] The causes of these complications are multifactorial, including an increase in the sympathetic nervous system in response to oxygen desaturations and arousals from sleep, free radical production from re-oxygenation, and large negative intrathoracic pressures that in turn increases the intramural pressure of vessels within the intrathoracic cavity. Additionally, OSA has clearly been shown to be related to the onset and recurrence of atrial fibrillation.[12]

OSA has also been linked with metabolic disorders.[13] New evidence suggests that untreated OSA is an independent risk factor for the development of Type 2 diabetes mellitus.[7]

Other risks of untreated OSA include depression, poor job performance, impaired family relationships, reduction in quality of life, and increased risk of motor vehicle accidents.

CLINICAL EVALUATION

Patients with OSA often present in clinic with an assortment of complaints related to nocturnal respiratory disturbances, fragmented sleep, and daytime sequelae. In other situations, patients may present not due to their own concern, but rather due to the concerns of a bed partner or family member.

Symptoms

In the evaluation of suspected sleep apnea, it is crucial to ascertain both nocturnal symptoms as well as those that occur during the day. In our experience, nocturnal symptoms are more reliably provided by a bed partner, and it is important to include the bed partner in the evaluation when possible.

Classic nighttime symptoms of OSA include:

- Loud Snoring: Frequently reported by bed partners, loud and disruptive snoring is a hallmark symptom of OSA due to upper airway obstruction during sleep.
- Witnessed Apneas: Partners or family members may observe episodes of breathing cessation or gasping during sleep, indicating significant airflow limitation.
- Excessive Daytime Sleepiness: Patients with OSA often experience excessive daytime sleepiness despite seemingly adequate nocturnal sleep, leading to impaired cognitive function, reduced productivity, and an increased risk of accidents or errors.
- Morning Headaches: Headaches upon awakening are commonly reported by individuals with OSA, attributed to nocturnal hypoxemia and hypercapnia leading to cerebral vasodilation and increased intracranial pressure.
- Nonrestorative Sleep: Patients may describe feeling unrefreshed or unrested despite spending an adequate duration in bed, reflecting disrupted sleep architecture and poor sleep quality.
- Nocturia: Frequent awakenings to urinate during the night, known as nocturia, are often reported by individuals with OSA.

Daytime symptoms of OSA include:

- Excessive daytime sleepiness: While it is the most common daytime symptom caused by OSA, it is important to recognize that many patients with diagnosed OSA do not report significant daytime sleepiness. Some studies have shown that less than 50% of patients with moderate to severe OSA have excessive daytime sleepiness.[5]
- Difficulty concentrating
- Memory difficulties
- Brain fog
- Irritability
- Hyperactivity
- Fatigue
- Drowsy driving.

Pediatric Considerations

In the pediatric population, daytime symptoms differ significantly from the adult population. At night, they similarly exhibit loud snoring or difficult breathing while asleep as well as significant sweating or restlessness at night.

During the daytime, particularly among younger pediatric patients, developmental, behavioral, and learning issues are most common. Many of the symptoms displayed may mimic those of attention deficit hyperactivity disorder.

Older children or teenagers may present with the symptoms of excessive daytime sleepiness, like adults.

Special attention should be paid to patients with Down syndrome or other neuromuscular disorders as there is a higher prevalence of OSA in these populations compared with the general pediatric population.[7]

Objective Tools to Use in Clinic

The Epworth Sleepiness Scale (**Box 1**) is an objective scale that is frequently used to assess the degree of sleepiness. A score higher than 10 indicates the patient is experiencing pathologic excessive daytime sleepiness.

A commonly used screening tool for OSA is the STOP-BANG score, which provides an objective tool to assess a patient's likelihood of having OSA.

The STOP-BANG mnemonic includes the following:

S: "Do you snore loudly, louder than talking, or enough to be heard through closed doors?"

T: "Do you feel tired or fatigued during the daytime almost every day?"

O: "Has anyone observed that you stop breathing during sleep?"

P: "Do you have a history of high blood pressure with or without treatment?"

B: BMI greater than 35 kg/m^2.

A: Age greater than 50 years.

N: Neck circumference greater than 43 cm (17 in).

G: Gender, male

The most recent 2017 guideline from the United States Preventive Services Task Force (USPSTF) states there is insufficient evidence to recommend the routine screening of OSA in asymptomatic patients.[14] Nevertheless, in patients where there is concern for

---

Box 1
Epworth Sleepiness Scale

How likely are you to doze off or fall asleep in the following situations, in contrast to feeling just tired? Use the following scale and indicate the most appropriate number for each situation. Answer choices for each situation range from 0 to 3. 0 = would never doze 1 = slight chance of dozing 2 = moderate chance of dozing 3 = high chance of dozing

Situation
  Sitting and Reading
  Watching TV
  Sitting, inactive in a public place (eg, a theater or meeting)
  As a passenger in a car for an hour without a break
  Lying down to rest in the afternoon when circumstances permit
  Sitting and talking with someone
  Sitting quietly after lunch without alcohol
  In a car, while stopped for a few minutes in traffic
  TOTAL (Range of 0–24)

OSA, the STOP-BANG score can be a helpful clinical tool to guide whether further testing or evaluation is warranted. An STOP-BANG score of 3 indicates an intermediate risk for moderate to severe OSA, whereas a score of 5 indicates a high risk for moderate to severe OSA. Specifically, with a score of 3 or higher, the sensitivity for OSA is 87% and the specificity for OSA is 31%.[5] The STOP-BANG tool can be accessed here.[15]

Risk Factors/Comorbid Medical Conditions

The major predisposing risk factor for OSA is excess body weight. In fact, it is estimated that ~60% of moderate to severe OSA is attributable to obesity.[7] In general, as the BMI increases, there is an increased risk of OSA. Among patients with morbid obesity, there is an extremely high prevalence of OSA.

Other risk factors to consider include middle-aged and older adults, postmenopausal status in women, patients with bony or soft structure abnormalities of the head and neck, endocrine disorders such as acromegaly or hypothyroidism, patients with Down syndrome or other neurologic disorders.

Patients who consume alcohol or sedating medications prior to bed are also at an increased risk of OSA.[7]

Physical Examination

The examination of patients with suspected OSA should include the following:
Anthropometric Measurements:

- BMI. BMI $\geq$ 30 kg/m^2, is a strong risk factor for OSA and contributes to airway narrowing and collapsibility
- Neck circumference. NC greater than 17 inches in men, 16 inches in women indicates an increased risk of OSA

Craniofacial Examination:

- Modified Mallampati Classification: This assesses the visibility of the oropharyngeal structures during phonation. Mallampati Scores of III and IV are associated with higher risk of upper airway obstruction.[16]
- Nasal patency: this can identify nasal obstruction that would contribute to mouth breathing. This in turn leads to an increased upper airway resistance during sleep.
- Oropharyngeal anatomy: Specific attention should be paid to tonsillar presence/size, uvula size, or whether the palate is high arching.
- Mandible: Position and size of the mandible should be assessed. Retrognathia and micrognathia are both associated with an increased risk of OSA.[5]
- Dentition: Quality and position of dentition as well as the presence of dentures should be assessed.
- Tongue size: Macroglossia is a common finding among patients with OSA. Patients with macroglossia may demonstrate scalloping of the tongue along the lateral edges.

Other important components of the physical examination:

- Cardiovascular examination: assess for murmurs or cardiac arrhythmias as well as edema or jugular venous distension as signs of heart failure.
- Pulmonary: assess for pulmonary vascular congestion.

TESTING OPTIONS FOR OBSTRUCTIVE SLEEP APNEA

OSA can only be diagnosed with objective testing. The primary testing options for OSA include nocturnal PSG and home sleep apnea testing (HSAT).

PSG is the gold standard for OSA diagnosis because it provides comprehensive monitoring of sleep architecture, respiratory parameters, as well as physiologic variables. Standard PSG monitoring includes electroencephalogram (EEG), facial electromyography (EMG), and electrooculogram (EOG), oronasal airflow, microphone for snoring or somniloquy, pulse oximetry, respiratory effort, body position, leg EMG, and single-lead electrocardiogram. While more thorough and comprehensive, patients may find laboratory testing to be more uncomfortable than their home environment, and this testing is significantly more expensive that HSAT.

HSAT is more accessible and cost-effective compared with PSG. It is reserved for those with high pretest probability for OSA and who lack comorbidities that would require an in-lab PSG. Examples of comorbidities that are a contraindication to HSAT include asthma, Chronic Obstructive Pulmonary Disease (COPD), CHF, comorbid sleep conditions, cognitive impairment, or morbid obesity (BMI >40 or 50). HSAT is generally more convenient for patients compared with in-laboratory PSG. HSAT options are numerous, and this is an area that continues to expand in terms of device options. Some HSAT options record oronasal airflow, respiratory effort, snore microphone, body position, and pulse oximetry. One newer HSAT option that has increased in use and popularity is the WatchPAT, which measures peripheral arterial tone to detect respiratory events and has no oronasal airflow monitoring. See **Table 1** for a summary of the comparison between PSG and HSAT options.

Overnight oximetry is sometimes used for screening purposes. While oximetry can give valuable insight into respiratory patterns or oxygen desaturation frequency during sleep, it is not capable of making a diagnosis of OSA and should not be used for diagnostic purposes.

Pediatric Considerations

In-laboratory PSG is currently the gold standard and only testing option to diagnose OSA in pediatrics populations. Current HSAT options are not approved or indicated for use in the pediatric population, and they should only have a PSG.[17]

DIAGNOSING OBSTRUCTIVE SLEEP APNEA

Regardless of testing type, all testing for OSA identifies the total number of abnormal respiratory events that occur for the duration of the night. Specifically, these events refer to the total number of apneas and hypopneas. An apnea is defined as a complete upper airway obstruction lasting for at least 10 seconds, whereas a hypopnea is defined as a partial upper airway obstruction lasting for at least 10 seconds and causing either an oxygen desaturation or arousal from sleep.[5,7,18] The total number of events is then divided by the number of hours of sleep. The result of this value is called the Apnea Hypopnea Index (AHI), and this is what is used to diagnose OSA. In adults, an AHI greater than 5 events per hour is considered diagnostic for OSA. See **Table 2** for how OSA severity is defined by the AHI in adults and **Table 3** for pediatrics. In the pediatric population, OSA is diagnosed if the AHI exceeds 1 event per hour.

TREATMENT OF OBSTRUCTIVE SLEEP APNEA

Numerous treatment options exist for OSA in adults and children, and they vary in both efficacy as well as patient convenience. The treatment of OSA requires frequent follow-up and close monitoring of response, and a patient-centered approach should always be prioritized.

Table 1
Diagnostic testing options for obstructive sleep apnea

Diagnostic Test	Description	Advantages	Limitations
Polysomnography (PSG)	Gold standard for OSA diagnosis; comprehensive assessment of sleep architecture, and respiratory parameters.	Provides detailed information on sleep stages, respiratory events, and physiologic variables including facial and limb electromyography, single-lead electrocardiogram.	More expensive than HSAT, requires overnight laboratory monitoring with a technician, may not be as readily accessible.
Home Sleep Apnea Testing (HSAT)	Portable monitoring devices used for out-of-center testing; simplified version of PSG with fewer parameters. Only used in patients with high pretest probability of OSA who lack significant comorbidities	Convenient, cost-effective, and accessible for patients; suitable for uncomplicated cases of OSA.	Limited ability to assess sleep architecture and comorbid sleep disorders; less comprehensive than PSG. May have reduced accuracy in patients with certain comorbidities.

Abbreviation: OSA, Obstructive sleep apnea.

Table 2
Obstructive sleep apnea severity by Apnea Hypopnea Index in adults

AHI	OSA Severity
0–4.9	Normal/none
5–14.9	Mild
15–29.9	Moderate
30 or higher	Severe

Abbreviations: AHI, Apnea Hypopnea Index; OSA, obstructive sleep apnea.

Positive Airway Pressure

Positive airway pressure (PAP) therapy is the mainstay of management of OSA in adults. PAP therapy works by maintaining upper airway patency by pressurizing the upper airway and thus prevents the collapse of the upper airway during sleep.

There are various types of PAP therapy that include CPAP, Automatically titration continuous positive airway pressure (Auto-CPAP), Bilevel positive airway pressure (BiPAP), noninvasive positive pressure ventilation, and adaptive servo ventilation. All PAP modalities are capable of detecting respiratory events including obstructive or central apneas as well as hypopneas. They report data including the AHI, average pressure used, and mask leak.

PAP therapy is recommended for all patients with moderate to severe range OSA and patients with mild OSA with significant daytime sleepiness.

Optimal PAP therapy is best identified with an in-laboratory titration PSG. In this study, the patient is placed on PAP therapy and various pressures and treatment modalities can be trialed until obstructive respiratory events resolve.

Sleep clinicians will frequently order a "split night" PSG. In this study, the first portion of the study is spent without the patient on no therapy and is used to diagnose OSA based on the criteria outlined above or based on criteria defined by insurance companies. If the patients meet the criteria for OSA, they are started on PAP therapy during the latter portion of the night to identify optimal PAP therapy. If optimal PAP therapy is not identified, they will then come back for a full night titration PSG.

Many patients diagnosed with OSA via HSAT are started on Auto-CPAP. This is a PAP modality that is programmed to provide a range of CPAP pressures. The machine will then detect airflow obstruction and increase the pressure to alleviate the obstruction. The benefit of Auto-PAP is that the patient avoids the inconvenience of an in-laboratory PSG. Pressures can be adjusted in follow-up appointments based on the data the machine reports back.

Common side effects of PAP therapy include mask leak, aerophagia, mask discomfort, claustrophobia, dry nose, and dry mouth.

Table 3
Obstructive sleep apnea severity by Apnea Hypopnea Index in children

AHI	OSA Severity
0–0.9	Normal/none
1–4.9	Mild
5–9.9	Moderate
10 or higher	Severe

Abbreviations: AHI, Apnea Hypopnea Index; OSA, obstructive sleep apnea.

Studies have shown PAP therapy to be effective in improving subjective symptoms of OSA. Of interest, studies examining improvements of objective measurements of OSA have not been as definitive. One aspect of PAP therapy that appears to denote subjective and objective benefit in patients with OSA is duration of treatment, with a usage of 7 hours or more showing significant improvement in both subjective and objective measurements.[5,19]

One of the main limitations of PAP therapy is nonadherence. Some studies show that after 1 year less than 50% of patients continue to use PAP therapy.[20] Other studies have shown that among patients who use CPAP regularly, the average use is only 58.7% of the total sleep time.[21] This is particularly problematic when one considers that the minimum number of hours of CPAP use per night needed to reap benefits from its use is between 5 and 6 hours per night. Numerous interventions have been implemented to attempt to increase PAP adherence including more comfortable therapy, new masks, and improved remote monitoring. While PAP therapy is first-line therapy for OSA, marked nonadherence is a significant barrier to management.

There is no generally accepted timeframe for when testing should be repeated. Common indications for repeat testing include persistent poor mask leak, aerophagia or discomfort with CPAP (for which BiPAP can be tried), worsened daytime sleepiness despite adequate PAP usage, persistent elevated leak or poor mask fit, or 10% weight loss or weight gain from the patient's weight at the time of their last study. Specifically, repeat testing for weight gain/loss is indicated to assess for a change in OSA severity or a need for increased or decreased PAP pressures.

Oral Appliances

The most effective oral appliance for the treatment of OSA is a mandibular advancement device (MAD). These are indicated for patients with mild to moderate OSA or patients with severe OSA that cannot tolerate PAP therapy. They work by protruding the mandible which in turn opens the airway by pulling the base of the tongue forward.

Patients who are most likely to benefit from a MAD include younger patients, patients with lower BMI, patients with positional (supine-dependent) OSA, and good dentition.[22] Patients with dentures are not candidates for MADs.

MADs should be fitted and managed by a dentist with sleep-specific training.

Patients who are using a MAD should undergo repeat testing once their device is felt to be at the optimal setting to determine whether OSA severity has been reduced by the MAD. Studies show the response to MAD in regards to OSA reduction to be more variable than with PAP therapy, and thus they should have close follow-up.[5]

Common side effects of MAD include temporomandibular joint dysfunction and chronic bite changes.

Hypoglossal Nerve Stimulator

In 2014, the FDA approved a novel therapy for OSA called Inspire. It is second-line therapy and can only be used or considered in patients who cannot tolerate PAP therapy. Inspire is a hypoglossal nerve stimulator. It is a permanently installed device that is implanted in the right side of the chest with leads that stimulate the hypoglossal nerve at the beginning of inspiration and causes tongue protrusion, which in turn brings the base of the tongue forward to open the airway.[5,23]

Inspire is currently approved for adult patients 18 years and older with an AHI of 15/h to 100/h with a BMI less than 40 kg/m^2. Additionally, patients must have less than 25% central respiratory events on sleep testing performed within the past 2 years. Prior to having the procedure, the patient must have consultation with an Inspire-trained otolaryngologist with a drug-induced sleep endoscopy to evaluate for concentric collapse, which is a contraindication to PAP therapy. More information on Inspire can be found here.[24]

Studies have shown that 70% of patients with Inspire maintain a reduction in their AHI of 50% or more and AHI less than 20/h over time.[5,25] Additionally, patients who have Inspire tend to use therapy more often and for longer durations compared with patients using CPAP.[26]

While certainly a welcome and beneficial therapy, it is important to emphasize that for now this remains a second-line treatment option.

Other Surgical Therapies

In some patients, there may be specific anatomic abnormalities that can be targeted surgically in efforts to treat OSA. Historically, uvulopalatopharyngoplasty (UPPP) was performed as a surgical treatment for OSA. Long-term studies have shown that the benefits of UPPP tend to decrease over time to less than 50%, and thus UPPP is only performed in specific situations as per the recommendation of otolaryngology.[27] As a general principle, in a patient with refractory OSA or obvious anatomic abnormalities, further assessment by otolaryngology is recommended.

Bariatric surgery is commonly performed in patients with OSA given the significant overlap between obesity and OSA as discussed previously. Most studies have shown a reduction in AHI and BMI after bariatric surgery, but this does not guarantee resolution of OSA. Repeat sleep testing should be performed once the patient reaches a steady weight after surgery.[5]

Other Treament Recommendations

Positional sleep therapy is a common treatment recommendation used often in conjunction with other treatment strategies in patients with OSA that worsens in the supine position. Positional devices are typically worn and prevent inadvertently rolling into the supine position. They are not usually covered by insurance.

Alcohol use should be monitored in all patients with OSA given that alcohol is known to worsen OSA severity. Specifically, alcohol use should be avoided within 2 to 4 hours of sleep.[28]

Similarly, clinicians should avoid prescribing sedating medications such as benzodiazepines and opioids to patients with untreated OSA.

Pediatric Considerations

In the pediatric population, first-line therapy for OSA is tonsillectomy and adenoidectomy (T&A). In patients with confirmed OSA, a referral to ENT for evaluation for T&A is recommended as the first step. If the surgery is performed, repeat testing 3 to 6 months after treatment is recommended to evaluate for the resolution of OSA. The Childhood Adenotonsillectomy Trial (CHAT) study found significant improvements in quality of life and polysomnographic findings in patients who underwent tonsillectomy.[29] Specifically, in children who underwent tonsillectomy, the AHI dropped from 4.8/h to 1.3/h compared with a drop from 4.5/h to 2.9/h in patients who had watchful waiting. Those who underwent tonsillectomy also saw improvements in the Pediatric Quality of Life Inventory compared with those who underwent watchful waiting with an increase of 5.9 from baseline versus an increase of 0.9, respectively.[29]

If OSA persists after tonsillectomy or if the patient is found to not be a candidate for surgery, CPAP or BiPAP can be used in pediatrics following similar principles to those used in the adult population.

Weight loss should be prioritized in pediatric patients with obesity as well.

SUMMARY

OSA is an underdiagnosed heterogeneous condition that affects adults and children. Diagnosis and management of OSA can lead to significant subjective improvement in patient's lives. Given the significant burden of disease as well as significant medical comorbidities, accurate and prompt recognition of OSA by primary care physicians with appropriate work-up and management is crucial.

CLINICS CARE POINTS

- Snoring and daytime sleepiness are key indicators of OSA in adults.
- Attention or behavioral issues in children should raise suspicion for possible OSA.
- Resistant hypertension should raise suspicion for possible OSA.
- Daytime sleepiness and fatigue may be misattributed to other medical conditions such as depression. OSA should be considered in the differential for these common complaints.
- OSA is underdiagnosed in women and in patients who lack classic clinical features.
- While home sleep testing is becoming more common, a negative home sleep test does not mean a patient does not have obstructive sleep apnea.
- Lifestyle and behavioral changes can significantly improve or resolve OSA and should always be included in the treatment plan.

DISCLOSURE

None.

REFERENCES

1. Burwell CS, Robin ED, Whaley RD, et al. Extreme obesity associated with alveolar hypoventilation—a Pickwickian syndrome. Obes Res 1994;2:390–7.
2. Anderson KN. Insomnia and cognitive behavioural therapy-how to assess your patient and why it should be a standard part of care. J Thorac Dis 2018; 10(Suppl 1).
3. ResMedica clinical newsletter. Available at: https://document.resmed.com/en-au/documents/articles/clinical_newsletter/resmedica14.pdf. Accessed January 28, 2024.
4. Rundo JV. Cleve Clin J Med 2019;86(9 Suppl 1):2–9.
5. Kryger, Meir H, et al. Chapter 131, obstructive sleep apnea: clinical features, evaluation, and principles of management, . Kryger's principles and practice of sleep medicine. 7th edition. Elsevier; 2022. p. 1244–59.
6. Andrisani G, Andrisani G. Sleep apnea pathophysiology. Sleep Breath 2023; 27(6):2111–22.
7. American Academy of Sleep Medicine. Obstructive Sleep Apnea Discrders. International classification of sleep disorders. 3rd edition. American Academy of Sleep Medicine; 2014. p. 53–68.
8. McNicholas WT, Pevernagie D. Obstructive sleep apnea: transition from pathophysiology to an integrative disease model. J Sleep Res 2022;31(4). https://doi.org/10.1111/jsr.13616.
9. Dempsey JA, Smith CA, Przybylowski T, et al. The ventilatory responsiveness to CO_2 below eupnoea as a determinant of ventilatory stability in sleep. J Physiol 2010;588(5):737–51.

10. Smith PL, Schwartz AR, Patil SP. Instabilities of the ventilatory control system in obstructive sleep apnea. Sleep 2019;42(7).
11. Terrill PI, Edwards BA, Nemati S, et al. Quantifying the ventilatory control contribution to sleep apnoea using polysomnography. Eur Respir J 2015;45(2):408–18.
12. Kryger, Meir H, et al. Chapter 146, cardiovascular effects of sleep-related breathing disorders, . Kryger's principles and practice of sleep medicine. 7th edition. Elsevier; 2022. p. 1430–9.
13. Kryger, Meir H, et al. Chapter 136, cardiovascular effects of sleep-related breathing disorders, . Kryger's principles and practice of sleep medicine. 7th edition. Elsevier; 2022. p. 1318–26.
14. U.S. Preventive Services Task Force. Obstructive sleep apnea in adults: screening [Internet]. U.S. Preventive Services Task Force 2024. Available at: https://www.uspreventiveservicestaskforce.org/uspstf/recommendation/obstructive-sleep-apnea-in-adults-screening.
15. STOP-BANG score for obstructive sleep apnea (OSA) [Internet]. MDcalc 2024. Available at: https://www.mdcalc.com/calc/3992/stop-bang-score-obstructive-sleep-apnea.
16. Ramachandran SK, Kheterpal S, Consens F, et al. Derivation and validation of a simple perioperative sleep apnea prediction score. Anesth Analg 2010;110(4):1007–15.
17. American Academy of Sleep Medicine. AASM releases position statement on home sleep apnea testing. 2017. Available at: https://aasm.org/aasm-releases-position-statement-home-sleep-apnea-testing/. Accessed May 20, 2024.
18. American Academy of Sleep Medicine. The AASM Manual for the Scoring of Sleep and Associated Events: Rules, Terminology and Technical Specifications. Darien, IL: American Academy of Sleep Medicine; 2023. Version 3.
19. Marklund M, Braem MJA, Verbraecken J. Update on oral appliance therapy. Eur Respir Rev 2019;28(153):190083.
20. Pataka A, Kotoulas SC, Gavrilis PR, et al. Adherence to CPAP treatment: can mindfulness play a role? Life 2023;13(2):296.
21. Rotenberg BW, Murariu D, Pang KP. Trends in CPAP adherence over twenty years of data collection: a flattened curve. J Otolaryngol Head Neck Surg 2016;45(1):43.
22. Inspire Medical Systems. Inspire therapy. Available at: https://professionals.inspiresleep.com/en-us/our-therapy/. Accessed May 31, 2024.
23. U.S. Food and Drug Administration. Inspire upper airway stimulation - P130008/S090. Accessed [insert access date]. Available at: https://www.fda.gov/medical-devices/recently-approved-devices/inspire-upper-airway-stimulation-p130008s090.
24. Strollo PJ Jr, Soose RJ, Maurer JT, et al. Upper-airway stimulation for obstructive sleep apnea. N Engl J Med 2014;370(2):139–49.
25. Thaler E, Schwab R, Maurer J, et al. Results of the ADHERE upper airway stimulation registry and predictors of therapy efficacy. Laryngoscope 2020;130(5):1333–8.
26. He M, Yin G, Zhan S, et al. Long-term efficacy of uvulopalatopharyngoplasty among adult patients with obstructive sleep apnea: a systematic review and meta-analysis. Otolaryngol Head Neck Surg 2019;161(3):401–11.
27. Simou E, Britton J, Leonardi-Bee J. Alcohol and the risk of sleep apnoea: a systematic review and meta-analysis. Sleep Med 2018;42:38–46.
28. Marcus CL, Moore RH, Rosen CL, et al, Childhood Adenotonsillectomy Trial CHAT. A randomized trial of adenotonsillectomy for childhood sleep apnea. N Engl J Med 2013;368(25):2366–76.
29. Marcus CL, Moore RH, Rosen CL, et al. A randomized trial of adenotonsillectomy for childhood sleep apnea. N Engl J Med 2013;368(25):2366–76. https://doi.org/10.1056/NEJMoa1215881.

Tinnitus

Parvathi Perumareddi, DO

KEYWORDS

- Auditory pathways • Hearing loss • Cochlear damage • Hearing aids
- Sound therapy • Acoustic neuroma • Loud sound exposure • Acoustic trauma

KEY POINTS

- Tinnitus is often seen in primary care offices but is challenging to manage.
- Tinnitus can affect a patient's quality of life.
- Although there are many potential causes of tinnitus, many cases are of unknown etiology.
- There is no gold standard in terms of curative treatment.
- Depending on cause, there are measures that may help improve living with tinnitus.

INTRODUCTION

Tinnitus, derived from the Latin word "tinnire," manifests as a perception of ringing or other sounds, such as "buzzing" or "hissing" in the ears without an obvious external source. It is a common symptom encountered by primary care physicians, with prevalence estimates in the United States ranging from 10% to 15%.[1,2] Tinnitus varies widely among individuals, presenting as unilateral or bilateral, with fluctuations in intensity and frequency that can be intermittent or continuous, lasting from a few minutes to being constant. It is not specific to any single disease and lacks a definitive pathophysiological mechanism, which complicates the identification of underlying causes. The severity of symptoms can range from mild irritation to significant distress.

Despite advancements in treatment, there is currently no known cure for tinnitus although it can be improved or sometimes remit depending on the etiology. When persistent, it often adversely affects quality of life for patients, potentially leading to psychological distress and impacting daily functioning. Moreover, tinnitus places a substantial burden on both clinical resources and health care economics. In 2023, it was reported as the most compensated service-connected disability among US veterans.[3]

This article highlights the pervasive nature of tinnitus, its impact on individuals, and current recommendations in management.

Department of Medicine, Schmidt College of Medicine- Florida Atlantic University, 777 Glades Road, Boca Raton, FL 33431, USA
E-mail address: pperumar@health.fau.edu

Prim Care Clin Office Pract 52 (2025) 61–70
https://doi.org/10.1016/j.pop.2024.09.008
0095-4543/25/© 2024 Elsevier Inc. All rights reserved, including those for text and data mining, AI training, and similar technologies.
primarycare.theclinics.com

INCIDENCE/PREVALENCE

According to the National Health Interview Survey, in 2014, the prevalence of tinnitus in the United States was 11.2% with a range of 10% to 15% in adults.[4] The rate may actually be higher as not all patients seek care for this. In this survey, the rates were higher among non-Hispanic Whites versus other ethnicities and men versus women. Prevalence is known to be higher in older adults with peak occurrence in the 60 to 69-year-old age group but the distribution between men and women is equal, although men report the symptom more often.[5] Some studies show that only 1 in 5 people may seek care at some point, which means the majority individuals with tinnitus may suffer in silence.[6–8]

CLASSIFICATIONS

Tinnitus is classified based on whether the sound is perceptible only to the patient (subjective tinnitus) or can be heard by someone else, typically a physician using a stethoscope (objective tinnitus). Subjective tinnitus is the most prevalent type and is often linked to damage along the auditory pathways. In contrast, objective tinnitus, occurring less frequently, typically originates from a mechanical source such as muscular or vascular. When the cause is related to muscular, it involves one of the ears, nose, and throat muscles and will often be described as "clicking" in nature, whereas, a vascular source due to turbulent blood flow will be pulsatile.[9] Further classification involves determining whether an underlying cause can be identified. Primary tinnitus refers to cases where no specific cause is known, often termed idiopathic. While primary tinnitus may be associated with sensorineural hearing loss (SNHL), this connection is not necessary. Patients with primary tinnitus often find this symptom frustrating due to the absence of identifiable pathology and its impact on their lives.

On the other hand, secondary tinnitus usually results from an identifiable underlying condition or etiology, although it occurs less frequently than primary tinnitus. Management of secondary tinnitus focuses on addressing the root cause contributing to the auditory perception.[4]

It is essential to note that these classifications may overlap: subjective and objective refer to the perception of sound, while primary and secondary describe whether an underlying cause can be determined. Understanding these distinctions aids in tailoring appropriate diagnostic and therapeutic strategies for patients affected by tinnitus.

ETIOLOGIES

The mechanism or pathophysiology of subjective tinnitus is not clearly understood and in fact may be due to more than 1 cause. Multiple studies suggest that the dysfunction being in the cochlea and then an imbalance of neural activity is generated in the central pathway with a resultant perception of the abnormal sound of tinnitus. If the auditory system is involved over a longer period of time in these patients, the limbic system becomes affected as does the autonomic nervous system. Depending on location of the abnormalities, secondary changes occur which are hypothesized to explain the differences in pitch and volume of the tinnitus over time.[10,11]

Hearing Loss

Subjective tinnitus tends to be associated with hearing loss (SNHL) without any other linked cause. Some studies denote tinnitus as a threshold phenomenon in which tinnitus arises from 1 factor, for example, chronic hearing loss and it becomes symptomatic upon the emergence of multiple trigger factors acting in a synergistic fashion.[12,13]

Noise Exposure

Data based on population studies reveal that loud noise exposure is one of the most common causes of tinnitus. Following noise exposure or trauma, the outer hair cells undergo temporary changes that increase gain in the central auditory system. Subsequently, the microstructures of the cochlea become damaged resulting in tinnitus. It is important to note that the environment stimulus can consist of either a single exposure to a loud noise/trauma or chronic exposure over time.[14]

Age

Tinnitus can occur if there is reduction in auditory function as a result of age or if there is an abnormal lesion in the auditory pathway as a result of aging. Presbycusis is linked to bilateral subjective tinnitus but because of the age representation (60–60 years), consideration should be given that there is a vascular component contributing as well. Hearing tends to regress at age 60, involving sensory loss of high- frequency sounds and tinnitus is most commonly found in this demographic, according to the American Tinnitus Association.[6,15]

Ototoxicity

There are a number of medications that have some association with tinnitus. When tinnitus occurs in conjunction with otoxicity from medications, it typically manifests as bilateral and subjective. While often transient and reversible upon stopping the drug, higher doses may result in permanent tinnitus.[16]
See **Fig. 1** – for medications associated with tinnitus.

Medical conditions

Tinnitus is not known to be pathognomonic for any 1 disease state but can occur in conjunction with other symptoms in an array of conditions, ranging from neurologic (head injury, schwannoma, multiple sclerosis, acoustic neuroma) to infectious (neurosyphilis, meningitis, otitis media) to other disorders (hypothyroidism, anemia, Lyme disease, idiopathic intracranial hypertension, arteriovenous malformation).[17–19]

Other relatively common associations include: presbycusis, chronic noise exposure, cerumen impaction and systemic hypertension.[16]

EVALUATION
History and Initial Assessment

It is important to discern what type of tinnitus the patient is experiencing, as some causes will warrant further evaluation acutely and maybe harmful, such as those due to critical conditions such as carotid dissection or severe trauma.[1] Classification begins via obtaining a thorough pertinent history with specific history questions and a focused physical examination.[20]

Once tinnitus is initially determined to not be emergent, it should be classified as pulsatile or non-pulsatile as this determines the potential causes affiliated with each. Pulsatile tinnitus, in which one perceives the tinnitus to be in synchronous with their heartbeat, tends to be less common than non-pulsatile with etiologies that include: systemic hypertension, vascular tumors, ateriovenous malformation, sinus venous thrombosis and idiopathic intracranial hypertension.[1,16]

Further delineation of non-pulsatile tinnitus involves determining whether or not hearing loss is present and finally, duration along with associated symptoms helps stratify.[1,16]

gentamicin
tobramycin
azithromycin
clarithromycin
doxycycline
chloroquine
quinine
ganciclovir
ribavirin

HPV vaccine
(bivalent & quadrivalent)
Pneumococcal polysaccharide

carbamazepine
pregabalin

bupivacaine
lidocaine
vecuronium

aspirin
NSAIDs
sulfasalazine

carboplatin
cisplatin
imatinib
capecitabine
paclitaxel

sidenafil

Miscellaneous

furosemide
torsemide

atorvastatin
bupropion
risedronate
varenicline
dopamine agonists
PPIs

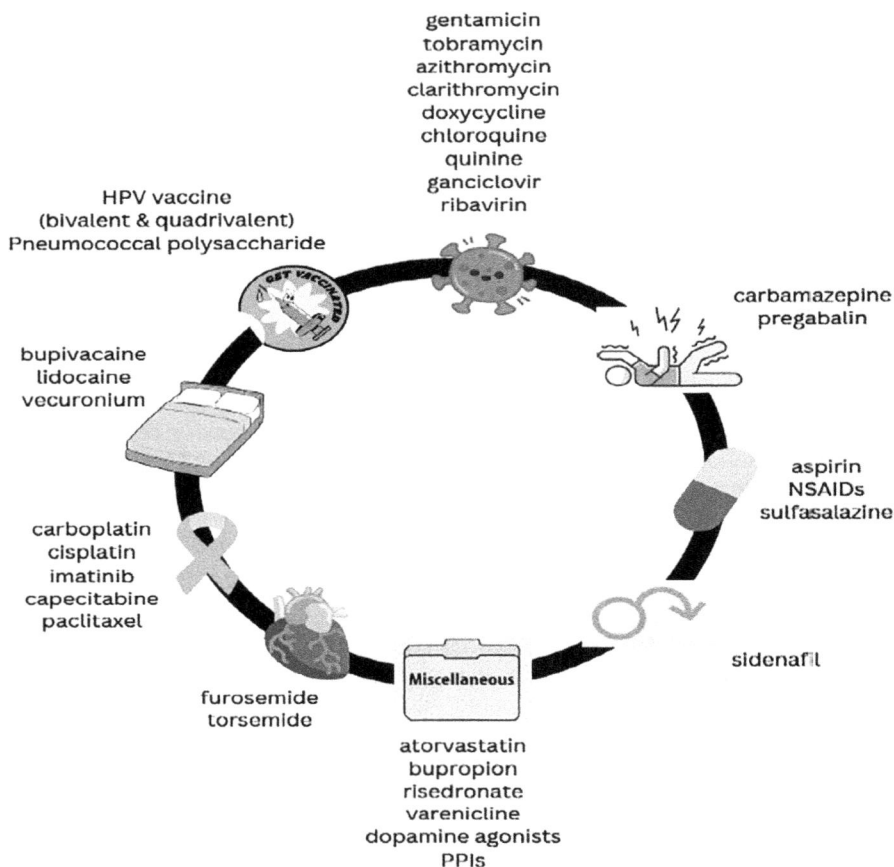

Fig. 1. Medications associated with Tinnitus.[20]

Severity is noted as "mild," "moderate," or "severe".

Location is assessed as "unilateral" or "bilateral" with the former signifying concern for structural lesions in the auditory region.

Duration is described as "acute" (<6 months) or chronic" (>6 months), with chronic being less likely to remit. In acute tinnitus, there may be an identifiable cause that is reversible.

Character should be noted and maybe described as "ringing" which is the classic quality but also might be "hissing" or "buzzing." These descriptions are typically associated with primary tinnitus whereas a "roaring" is usually indicative of a secondary cause.

Pulsatile or rhythmic clicking are both associated with neurologic conditions and warrant prompt referral. Also, if the tinnitus varies with change in physical activity or position, this can be related to neuro or vascular etiology.

Past medical history should be assessed for factors such as noise exposure, which can be occupational or social, acoustic trauma or injury, and medication use.

Finally, the presence (or absence of) associated symptoms should always be ascertained. These includes hearing loss, vertigo, ear pain, ear drainage, and imbalance as well as any that related to suspected differential diagnoses.[21]

Validated questionnaires were developed to evaluate the disabling consequences of tinnitus and that can be used to determine impact of the symptom for use in the clinical setting and/or in the research arena. These consist of Tinnitus Handicap Inventory (for clinical trials), Tinnitus Reaction Questionnaire, Tinnitus Functional Index, and Tinnitus Primary Functions Questionnaire.[22] Using these tools helps to distinguish between bothersome and non-bothersome tinnitus, with the latter not having a great impact on the quality of life and not requiring intervention.

It is vital to identify and treat concomitant disorders such as anxiety and depression as they can further impact quality of life in patients with tinnitus.[1]

Physical examination

A focused physical examination including head, eyes, ears, nose, and throat should be performed; neurologic, cardiovascular, vascular, and musculoskeletal are the important systems that should be assessed as key findings may potentially lead to source of tinnitus.

Key findings in physical exam that may aid in diagnosis include:

- Cerumen impaction
- Foreign body
- Otitis (media or externa)
- Nystagmus
- Papilledema
- Visual field defects
- Ataxia
- Carotid bruit

From the above, cerumen impaction, foreign body and otitis infections are potentially treatable and may alleviate the tinnitus. The rest warrant further investigation.[16]

There is also a grading scheme that can help delineate subjectively the degree of tinnitus the patient is experiencing in terms of impact on life.[1] See **Fig. 2** for- Grading scheme.

Diagnostic Studies

As mentioned previously, the majority of cases of tinnitus are primary or idiopathic and can be associated with SNHL in which case, an audiological examination is suggested.

In cases of secondary tinnitus, the goal is to identify the etiology and treat based upon the primary diagnosis. Depending on history and physical examination findings, this will guide what tests might be conducted.[16]

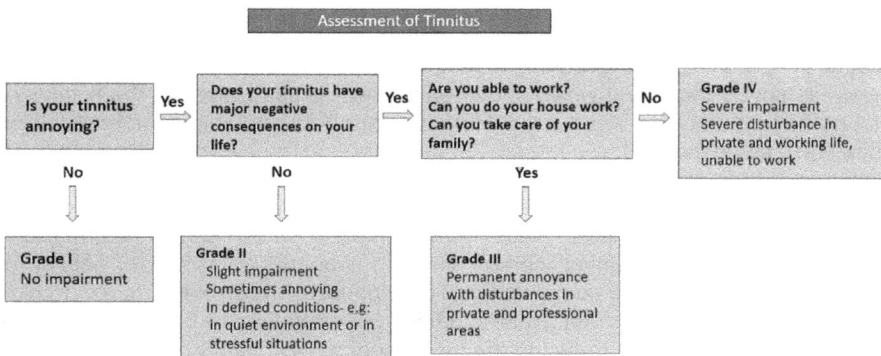

Fig. 2. Grading tinnitus.[1]

Referral for audiological examination should be performed in the following situations:

- Tinnitus accompanied by hearing loss,
- Persistent tinnitus (defined as longer than 6 months' duration),
- Unilateral tinnitus.

This evaluation determines if there is hearing loss as well as its severity and symmetry and dictates whether further testing is warranted such as auditory brainstem response test, high-frequency audiometry, or otoacoustic emissions test.[23]

As far as testing after hearing evaluation, specifically to measure the patient's subjective perception of the tinnitus, the audiologist may test the following:[24]

- Tinnitus sound matching—pitch and sounds are layered to match the audio or recreate the patient's tinnitus to provide a baseline measure,
- Minimum masking level—volume is used to determine the where the narrowband noise masks the tinnitus to provide a measure of how loud the patient senses the tinnitus,
- Loudness discomfort level—volume is used to determine when the sound becomes irritating for the patient which informs the likelihood of treatments such as masking, sound therapy, and hearing aids helping.

MANAGEMENT

While there is no known cure for subjective tinnitus, management is aimed at prevention and mitigating the symptom to ameliorate the perception to improve quality of life. Medications have not been shown to be helpful in managing tinnitus and are therefore, not recommended.[22] Non-pharmacological methods used to lessen the symptom of tinnitus consist of the following:

Cognitive Behavioral Therapy

Cognitive Behavioral Therapy (CBT) has been found in several studies to be an effective method in some to reduce the severity and intrusiveness of the distress associated with tinnitus. Further, it was also helpful in mitigating mood-related symptoms such as insomnia.[25] Patients may develop negative emotions surrounding the tinnitus and as a result may feel anxious or depressed due to fear. CBT serves to dispel negative beliefs and behaviors and additionally to teach the patient how to develop positive coping mechanisms.[26] Sessions typically are advised with a professional to last between 8 and 24 weeks.[27]

Sound Therapy

Another method that has become more widely used to treat subjective tinnitus is known as sound therapy in which sound enrichment is used to mask the tinnitus or disrupt the neural activity which results from tinnitus. This can be accomplished using white noise machines or music therapy. In the latter, music is used to affect the cerebral cortex which reduces the tinnitus. The benefit of this tool is that it is non-invasive and easy which is appealing to patients. Music therapy is divided into non-customized and customized, with the latter including techniques such as hearing aids, masking therapy, and tinnitus retraining therapy. Hearing aids can be especially helpful for those individuals who have some extent of hearing loss. These methods aim to hide the tinnitus sensation or distract by using other types of sounds be it music or environmental ones with a goal of reducing the psychological reactions that are triggered in tinnitus.[28]

Patients who are candidates for cochlear implants commonly have tinnitus, from 68% to 86%, but a significant percentage (34%–92%) report improvement or resolution of tinnitus post cochlear implant.[27]

Sleep Hygiene

Patients with tinnitus often report difficulties with sleep which can be linked to the disturbing nature of the symptom but also to the worry associated with it. Sleep hygiene is one key area that can be emphasized to address concomitant insomnia. These tips include the customary ones affiliated with good sleep practice as follows:

- Go to bed and awake at same time daily.
- Avoid caffeine, smoking, alcohol, and heavy meals within 2 hours of bedtime.
- Set sleep environment as far as darkness (no blue light, devices, tv) and ambient temperature.
- Avoid exercise or stimulating activity (stress) 2 hours prior to bedtime.

CURRENT RESEARCH TOPICS
Deep Brain Stimulation

Some limited research with few cases shows a potential role for the use of deep brain stimulation (DBS) in the management of tinnitus. In DBS, electrodes are implanted in specific regions of the brain, the auditory cortex, caudate, and the thalamus, with the purpose of modulating neural activity in places of abnormality function. The limitation is the lack of randomized controlled trials as well as the small number of studies, however, despite very limited numbers, there was a positive outcome noted in 7 patients.[25]

Other topics of research including electrical suppression or stimulation such as transcranial magnetic stimulation (TMS) and bimodal stimulation have been studied but these have not been proven to be effective as treatment at this time.[20]

PATIENT EDUCATION POINTS

- Tinnitus is a symptom but not a disease.
- Exposure to loud noise can cause temporary tinnitus but chronic noise exposure can result in irreversible tinnitus, so caution should be exercised to avoid acoustic trauma for prevention of tinnitus.
- Tinnitus may occur in conjunction with hearing loss but not always.
- Options for management include non-invasive tools including CBT, sound therapy, hearing aids.
- There are professional organizations (such as American Tinnitus Association) created to help support patients with tinnitus.

SUMMARY

Tinnitus is a symptom affecting up to 15% of the population, maybe more, and although it varies in duration, intensity, and character, it can be quite bothersome and debilitating for patients. Evaluation consists of determining the type of tinnitus and working up based on whether subjective or objective, the latter of which is typically associated with a discrete medical condition.

Patient education and support is the cornerstone of family medicine. Best practices can go a long way to helping patients suffering from tinnitus.

While there is no cure for tinnitus, various options such as CBT, self-help resources (books, support groups), hearing aids, and sound therapy can offer some level of amelioration or coping in patients who experience bothersome tinnitus.

CASE STUDY

The patient is a 53-year-old male who works at a construction site for the past 20 years. Although he uses ear protection, he does have chronic exposure to loud machinery noises. He presents with complaint of persistent ringing in his ears which he first noticed 6 months ago. The symptom is noted to be bilateral and continuous and particularly noticeable in quiet environments.

Initial assessment included audiometric evaluation consisting of pure tone audiometry which revealed bilateral high-frequency sensorineural hearing loss. Tinnitus pitch was matched to 6000 Hz. Diagnosis of noise-induced hearing loss and noise-induced tinnitus was made. A treatment plan was formulated as follows

- Fitting with bilateral hearing aids programmed to amplify high-frequency sounds,
- Sound therapy was instituted in the form of built-in tinnitus masking in the hearing aids with white noise to mask the tinnitus,
- Counseling was provided to educate patient on the use of the hearing aids as well as the importance of consistently using hearing protection in loud environments.

Outcome: The patient returned for follow-up and noted a definite reduction in perception of tinnitus. Long-term prognosis yields expectation of maintained reduction of tinnitus with continuous use of hearing aids and compliance with hearing protection procedures.

CLINICS CARE POINTS

Based on summary of guideline action statements, the following are recommended:

- Perform a thorough focused history and physical examination, distinguishing between bothersome and non-bothersome tinnitus,
- Ascertain medications and drug-drug interactions that could be contributory,
- Obtain a prompt comprehensive audiology examination in patients with unilateral, persistent tinnitus, or hearing loss,
- Provide education for the patient on management strategies, including discussion on natural history,
- Offer cognitive behavioral therapy for patients with persistent, bothersome tinnitus.

The following do not have evidenced-based theory and are NOT recommended:

- Imaging studies unless indicated based on other co-existent symptoms such as focal neurologic abnormalities or in the case, pulsatile tinnitus or unilateral hearing loss,
- Pharmacotherapy such as anxiolytics, antidepressants, anticonvulsants,
- Herbals or dietary supplements such as ginkgo biloba,
- Transcranial magnetic stimulation (TMS).

DISCLOSURE

The author has no affiliations or funding to declare.

REFERENCES

1. Langguth B, Kreuzer PM, Kleinjung T, et al. Tinnitus: causes and clinical management. Lancet Neurol 2013;12(9):920–30.
2. Makar SK. Etiology and Pathophysiology of tinnitus - a systematic review. Int Tinnitus J 2021;25(1):76–86.
3. Batts S, Stankovic KM. Tinnitus prevalence, associated characteristics, and related healthcare use in the United States: a population-level analysis. Lancet Reg Health Am 2024;29:100659.
4. Baguley D, McFerran D, Hall D. Tinnitus. Lancet 2013;382(9904):1600–7.
5. Bhatt JM, Lin HW, Bhattacharyya N. Prevalence, severity, exposures, and treatment patterns of tinnitus in the United States. JAMA Otolaryngol Head Neck Surg 2016;142(10):959–65.
6. Shargorodsky J, Curhan GC, Farwell WR. Prevalence and characteristics of tinnitus among US adults. Am J Med 2010;123(8):711–8.
7. Henry JA, Dennis KC, Schechter MA. General review of tinnitus: prevalence, mechanisms, effects, and management. J Speech Lang Hear Res 2005;48(5):1204–35.
8. Henry JA, Griest S, Zaugg TL, et al. Tinnitus and hearing survey: a screening tool to differentiate bothersome tinnitus from hearing difficulties. Am J Audiol 2015;24(1):66–77.
9. Chan Y. Tinnitus: etiology, classification, characteristics, and treatment. Discov Med 2009;8(42):133–6. PMID: 19833060.
10. Henry JA, Roberts LE, Caspary DM, et al. Underlying mechanisms of tinnitus: review and clinical implications. J Am Acad Audiol 2014;25(1):5–22, quiz 126.
11. Atik A. Pathophysiology and treatment of tinnitus: an elusive disease. Indian J Otolaryngol Head Neck Surg 2014;66(Suppl 1):1–5.
12. Kujawa SG, Liberman MC. Adding insult to injury: cochlear nerve degeneration after "temporary" noise-induced hearing loss. J Neurosci 2009;29(45):14077–85.
13. Lanting CP, de Kleine E, van Dijk P. Neural activity underlying tinnitus generation: results from PET and fMRI. Hear Res 2009;255(1–2):1–13.
14. Mirz F, Gjedde A, Sødkilde-Jrgensen H, et al. Functional brain imaging of tinnitus-like perception induced by aversive auditory stimuli. Neuroreport 2000;11(3):633–7.
15. Roberts LE, Eggermont JJ, Caspary DM, et al. Ringing ears: the neuroscience of tinnitus. J Neurosci 2010;30(45):14972–9.
16. Dalrymple S, Lewis S, Philman S. Tinnitus: diagnosis and management. Am Fam Physician 2021;103(11):663–71.
17. Esmaili AA, Renton J. A review of tinnitus. Aust J Gen Pract 2018;47(4):205–8.
18. Wang H, Stern JI, Robertson CE, et al. Pulsatile tinnitus: differential diagnosis and approach to management. Curr Pain Headache Rep 2024. https://doi.org/10.1007/s11916-024-01263-1.
19. Tunkel DE, Bauer CA, Sun GH, et al. Clinical practice guideline: tinnitus. Otolaryngol Head Neck Surg 2014;151(2 Suppl):S1–40.
20. Wu V, Cooke B, Eitutis S, et al. Approach to tinnitus management. Can Fam Physician 2018;64(7):491–5.
21. Cima RFF, Mazurek B, Haider H, et al. A multidisciplinary European guideline for tinnitus: diagnostics, assessment, and treatment. HNO 2019;67(suppl 1):10–42.
22. Bauer CA. Tinnitus. N Engl J Med 2018;378(13):1224–31.
23. Fournier P, Cuvillier AF, Gallego S, et al. A new method for assessing masking and residual inhibition of tinnitus. Trends Hear 2018;22. 2331216518769996.

24. Basner L, Smit JV, Zeitler DM, et al. Deep brain stimulation for primary refractory tinnitus: a systematic review. Brain Sci 2024;14(5):452.
25. Chhaya V, Patel D, Shethia F, et al. Current therapeutic trends for tinnitus cure and control: a scoping review. Indian J Otolaryngol Head Neck Surg 2023;75(4):1–9.
26. Aazh H, Landgrebe M, Danesh AA, et al. Cognitive behavioral therapy for alleviating the distress caused by tinnitus, hyperacusis and misophonia: current perspectives. Psychol Res Behav Manag 2019;12:991–1002.
27. Park KW, Kullar P, Malhotra C, et al. Current and emerging therapies for chronic subjective tinnitus. J Clin Med 2023;12(20):6555.
28. Mi T, Qinxiu Z, Jie W. Music therapy for tinnitus: a systematic review and meta-analysis. Am J Otolaryngol 2024;45(5):104362.

Hearing Loss
Unmet Needs in a Digital Age

Tajwar Taher, MD[a],*, Frances Wu, MD[b]

KEYWORDS

- Hearing • Loss • Primary • Care • Differential • Diagnosis • Geriatric • Disparities

KEY POINTS

- Hearing loss occurs in all ages, but it is associated with a 20% mortality increase in the elderly.
- The etiology is often an accumulation of individual and environmental factors.
- Reducing noise exposure and timely intervention can significantly reduce disability.
- Digital tools on smartphones can help in resource-limited settings.
- Provider-dependent factors influence hearing disparities: failure to address hearing loss negatively impacts management of other health conditions.

INTRODUCTION AND BACKGROUND

Approximately 40 million adults (15.5%) in the US report difficulties hearing.[1,2] Sixty-five percent of adults aged over 60 years experience hearing loss, which bears a 20% mortality increase due to social withdrawal and isolation, distress, dementia, lost productivity from early retirement, costs of care, mental and physical declines, and poorer quality of life.[3] Hearing loss is also common in children and teens, affecting about 1 in 5 by the time they are 18 years of age. The prevalence of hearing loss doubles every decade from the age of 20 to 80 years.[1,4]

Only about 15% of adults with hearing loss use hearing aids.[3] Unaddressed hearing loss negatively impacts patients physically, mentally, socially,[5] and financially. As the third largest source of "years lived with disability" globally, the health care costs, educational support, lost productivity, and societal costs of hearing loss amount to about US$980 billion annually worldwide.[6]

Primary care providers (PCPs) are uniquely positioned to identify and address hearing loss. However, only about half of PCPs are comfortable formally identifying it.[7] Many lack the knowledge to evaluate it, face time constraints, and believe that it is

[a] Department of Family Medicine, Willamette Valley Medical Center, 2700 Southeast Stratus Avenue, McMinnville, OR 97128, USA; [b] Family Medicine Residency Program, Department of Family Medicine, Rutgers-RWJUH Somerset, 128 Rehill Avenue, Somerville, NJ 08876, USA
* Corresponding author.
E-mail address: taj.taher16@gmail.com

Prim Care Clin Office Pract 52 (2025) 71–85
https://doi.org/10.1016/j.pop.2024.09.009 **primarycare.theclinics.com**

detected through conversation alone, that high hearing aid costs preclude interventions, and that short life expectancy excludes benefitting from hearing support. Although the United States Preventative Services Task Force (USPSTF) gives hearing screening a grade I for older adults,[8] PCPs should still address hearing loss given its significant impact on quality of life. In this review, we aim to equip PCPs with the basic anatomy and pathophysiology of hearing loss, the tools available for the assessment in primary care, preventative guidance, effective treatments, and an awareness of social determinants in hearing loss.

DEFINITIONS

Hearing loss is categorized based on impairment, activity limitation, and social restriction, per the World Health Organization (WHO) and the International Classification of Functioning, Disability, and Health (**Table 1**). WHO grades can help clinicians understand the extent of disability and whether interventions are beneficial.

Hearing loss is further classified by mechanism. *Conductive hearing loss* refers to problems within the outer or middle ear, which prevent sound wave transmission to the inner ear. The outer ear consists of the external structures of the ear and canal up to the tympanic membrane. The middle ear begins with the tympanic membrane, which attaches to the 3 bones that conduct sound to the inner ear: the malleus, incus, and stapes.

Sensorineural hearing loss results from loss of function or damage to the inner ear (cochlea, semicircular canals, and stria vascularis) or the vestibulocochlear nerve (cranial nerve [CN] VIII). In the aging US population, presbycusis is the most prevalent form, involving death of the inner ear hair cells and metabolic derangements in the stria vascularis.

Mixed hearing loss refers to a combination of conductive and sensorineural hearing loss, while defects in neuronal transmission from CN VIII back to the auditory cortex of the superior temporal lobe result in the inability to interpret auditory input. This hearing loss is a defect in *central auditory processing* (**Fig. 1**).

ETIOLOGY

Hearing loss is not the inevitable result of the aging process; it arises from a combination of genetic factors, medical comorbidities, lifestyle, and environmental effects. Many factors affect individuals of every age: smoking, secondhand smoke, cerumen impaction, trauma, and nutritional deficiencies (vitamin A, zinc), viral infections, and environmental hazards. Some etiologies only occur in certain ages. It is helpful, therefore, to narrow the differential by stratifying patients by age. **Table 2** displays common causes of hearing loss by age and mechanism.

In the perinatal period, genetic disorders account for about 50% of cases. Many syndromes can impair ear structures from properly forming or functioning. The toxoplasmosis, other (zika, syphillis, mumps, parvovirus), Rubella, Cytomegalovirus, Herpes Simplex or HIV (TORCH) infections (particularly cytomegalovirus [CMV], herpes simplex virus [HSV] 1 and 2, Rubella, and Zika) may result in damage to the inner ear from inflammation, edema, and the presence of viral antigens. Low birth weight and maternal conditions such as pre-eclampsia have been associated with hearing loss, as well as neonatal hyperbilirubinemia and low activity, pulse, grimace, appearance, respiration (APGAR) scores.

A common transient cause of conductive hearing loss in childhood is otitis media. Due to the lack of studies with consistent findings, no conclusions about the relationship between hearing loss and recurrent or chronic otitis media can be made.[9] There

Table 1
World Health Organization grades

Grade	Hearing Threshold (dB)	Difficulty Hearing in Quiet Environments	Difficulty Hearing in Noisy Environments
Normal	<20	None	None to minimal
Mild	20 to <35	None with conversational speech	May have difficulty with conversational speech
Moderate	35 to <50	May have difficulty with conversational speech	Difficulty hearing and participating in conversation
Moderately severe	50 to <65	Difficulty hearing and participating in conversation	Difficulty hearing most speech and participating in conversation
Severe	65 to <80	Does not hear most conversational speech; may have difficulty hearing and understanding raised voices	Extreme difficulty hearing speech and participating in conversation
Profound	80 to <95	Extreme difficulty hearing raised voices	Conversational speech cannot be heard
Deafness	95 or greater	Cannot hear speech and most environmental sounds	Cannot hear speech and most environmental sounds
Unilateral	<20 in better ear, 35 or greater in affected ear	May not have problem unless sound is near affected ear. May have difficulty locating sounds	May have difficulty hearing speech and participating in conversations, or locating sounds

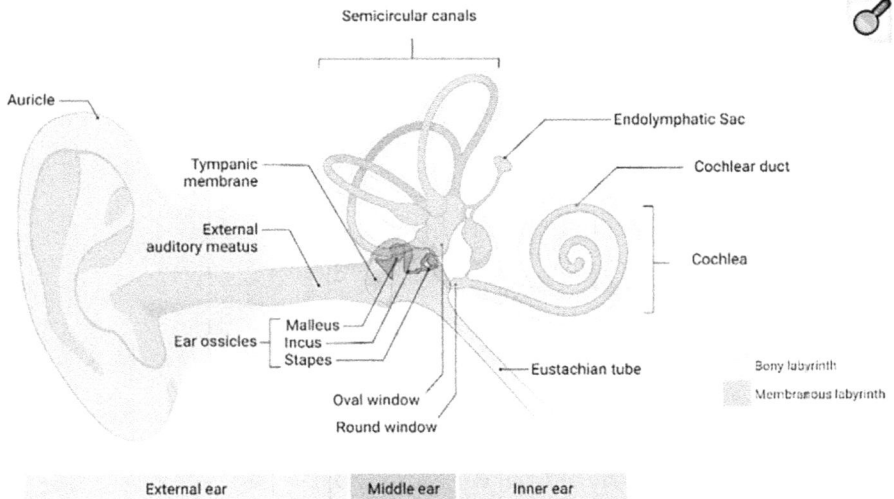

Fig. 1. The anatomy of the human ear includes the external, middle, and inner ear (comprising the cochlea and vestibular system). Created with BioRender.com. (*Data from* Khorrami M, Pastras C, Haynes PA, Mirzaei M, Asadnia M. The Current State of Proteomics and Metabolomics for Inner Ear Health and Disease. Proteomes. 2024 Jun 4;12(2):17. doi: 10.3390/proteomes12020017. PMID: 38921823; PMCID: PMC11207525.)

have been rare cases documented of severe otitis media resulting in meningitis with permanent hearing loss.[10]

For adults, common medical causes of hearing loss include chronic diseases (hypertension and diabetes), abnormal bone remodeling (otosclerosis), and presbycusis.[11] However, the greatest modifiable risk factor for acquired hearing loss is loud noise, usually from occupational exposures above 80 dB daily for greater than 40 weeks. The occupations with the most noise exposure include construction and landscaping, transportation (such as airport ground staff), work involving loud music or entertainment, agriculture, and other occupations involving loud machinery.[12] However, individuals are often exposed to loud noise even at home. The typical volume range for individuals listening to their personal devices is between 75 and 105 dB. About 50% of people aged 12 to 35 years listen to music too loudly by these standards.

Another major preventable risk factor is medications. Medications enter the endolymph of the inner ear, entering hair cells via passive diffusion, transporter channels, or endocytosis. Inner ear hair cells are among the few types of cell unable to actively clear ototoxins, leading to drug-mediated toxicities. Known ototoxic medications include aminoglycosides and cyclodextrins (incorporated in aripiprazole, ziprasidone, and voriconazole).[13] Certain medications that may not cause ototoxicity alone can do so when administered with others (eg, pancuronium and loop diuretics). Any systemic process that reduces clearance (renal insufficiency, depletion of antioxidants, fever, infection, transient ischemia, or hypoxia) increases the odds of ototoxicity. **Table 3** provides a list of common ototoxic medications.

Outer and inner hair cells cannot be regenerated. The spiral ganglia—which transmit the sensory input from the hair cells to CN VIII—cannot be bypassed if damaged, even with the insertion of cochlear implants. Vigilance about ototoxicity is, therefore, critical in any specialty.

Table 2
Differential diagnosis: age and mechanism

	Perinatal	Childhood/Adolescence	Adult/Elderly	All Ages
Conductive	Genetic: CHARGE, Stickler, and Apert syndromes	Otitis media with effusion	Otosclerosis Cholesteatoma Nasopharyngeal tumors	Cerumen impaction Trauma/iatrogenic
Sensorineural	TORCH infections, Hypoxia, Prematurity Genetic syndromic conditions (Waardenburg, Usher, Pendred, Jervell and Lange-Nielsen, and Alport)	—	Presbycusis Meniere's Diabetes Vestibular schwannoma Autoimmune (rheumatoid, lupus, and Wegener's)	Ototoxic medications Noise exposure Viral infections (HIV, HSV, and West Nile) Meningitis
Mixed	—	—	—	Noise exposure Trauma Infections
Central	Hyperbilirubinemia	Meningitis	Stroke	Zinc, Iron, Vitamin A deficiency

Table 3
Ototoxic medications

Class	Examples
Chemotherapeutics	Cisplatin, vincristine
Antibiotics	Aminoglycosides (gentamicin and neomycin)
	Macrolides
	Quinolones
	Vancomycin
	Imipenem + cilastin
Antivirals	Ganciclovir, ribavirin + interferon
Antifungals	Amphotericin
Antimalarials	Chloroquine and mefloquine
Analgesics	Aspirin and NSAIDs
Cardiac	Loop diuretics, acetazolamide, beta blockers, ramipril
Neurologic	Depakote and entacapone
Immunosuppressants	Tacrolimus and hydroxychloroquine

CLINICAL HISTORY

A detailed history is essential in determining the type, severity, and potential interventions for hearing loss. In most infants, universal hearing screening catches hearing impairments. Monitoring language and functional developmental milestones can further elucidate abnormal hearing.[14,15] In many cases, family members who have experienced difficulty communicating with patients are the ones to raise the alarm. Other findings include having to increase the volume on devices, frequently asking for repetition, social avoidance, and difficulty in noisy spaces or with background noise. Decreased hearing may also present with sensitivity to loud noises, tinnitus, or vertigo. Presbycusis classically presents with bilateral hearing loss, with difficulty recognizing speech regardless of the environment.

Causes of sudden onset unilateral hearing loss include Meniere's disease, vestibular schwannoma, autoimmune diseases, trauma, viral infections (coronavirus disease 2019), and vascular impairments. Providers should ask about common risk factors: noise exposure (both recreational and environmental), ototoxic medications, ear infections, cotton tip use for ear cleaning, diabetes mellitus, stroke, vasculitis, head or ear trauma, and family history.

Lastly, the American Academy of Otolaryngology–Head and Neck Surgery's 10 "Red Flags" for hearing loss[16] can help determine when urgent referral is warranted.

1. Hearing loss with a positive history of ear infections, noise exposure, familial hearing loss, tuberculosis, syphilis, HIV/AIDS, Meniere's disease, autoimmune disorder, ototoxic medication use, otosclerosis, von Recklinghausen's neurofibromatosis, and Paget's disease of bone, ear, or head trauma related to onset.
2. History of pain, active drainage, or bleeding from an ear.
3. Sudden onset or rapidly progressive hearing loss.
4. Acute, chronic, or recurrent episodes of dizziness.
5. Evidence of congenital or traumatic deformity of the ear.
6. Visualization of blood, pus, cerumen plug, foreign body, or other material in the ear canal.
7. An unexplained conductive hearing loss or abnormal tympanogram.

8. Unilateral or asymmetric hearing loss (a difference of >15 dB pure tone average between ears) or bilateral hearing loss greater than 30 dB.
9. Unilateral or pulsatile tinnitus.
10. Unilateral or asymmetrically poor speech discrimination scores (a difference of >15% between ears) or bilateral speech discrimination scores of less than 80%.

EVALUATION

The physical examination is the next step in evaluation. For infants and children, findings associated with genetic syndromes include heterochromia of the irises, malformations of the auricle or ear canal, dimpling or skin tags around the auricle, cleft lip or palate, asymmetry, hypoplasia of the facial structures, and microcephaly.[15]

Otoscopic inspection of the external auditory canal will reveal cerumen impaction, foreign objects, canal edema, erythema, and otorrhea. Cerumen impaction is particularly important to check for in patients with intellectual disabilities as they may not be able to express concerns about their hearing impairment or participate in subjective hearing tests. In fact, the prevalence of cerumen impaction in this population has been found to be 20%, compared to the 2% in the general population.[17]

The tympanic membrane should be inspected for its color, presence of bulging, perforation, and absence of normal landmarks such as the cone of light, handle of the malleus, umbo, pars tensa, and pars flaccida. Typically, the tympanic membrane is gray-colored and variably translucent, which allows for visualization of the incus and stapes. With pneumatic otoscopy, the normal tympanic membrane concaves to applied air pressure; this finding can confirm resolution of otitis media, while a flat tympanogram may signify effusion or perforation[18] (**Figs 2** and **3**).

The Weber and Rinne tests can distinguish unilateral causes of hearing loss.[19,20] The 512 Hz tuning fork is preferred as the 128 Hz and 256 Hz forks tend to vibrate more and confound results. To perform the Weber test, the tuning fork is struck one-third of the way down from the open end and placed on a bony surface of the face. For individuals with normal hearing, the sound will remain midline. For individuals with unilateral sensorineural hearing loss, the sound is heard better in the unaffected ear.[19] The Rinne test determines how air conduction compares to bone conduction. The tuning fork is struck, held next to the external canal, and then placed on the mastoid prominence. For individuals with unilateral sensorineural hearing loss, air conduction is better than bone conduction.

In the case of unilateral conductive hearing loss, the Weber test shows better hearing on the affected side. This is due to the masking effect, in which the mechanical obstruction in the ear masks the background noise in the air and allows for improved air conduction to the affected ear. The Rinne test shows better bone conduction than air conduction in the affected ear, with better air conduction than bone conduction in the unaffected ear.[20]

The whispered voice, watch tick, and finger rub tests have questionable accuracy and are largely operator dependent. They are not recommended as sole methods of evaluation.

Pure tone audiometry (PTA) remains the gold standard for diagnosis. Each ear can be tested individually, whereas in a sound booth (for people who cannot tolerate headphones, like children), the test cannot distinguish unilateral from bilateral hearing loss. PTA can also be adjusted to test toddlers and children through visual reinforcement and conditioned play protocols. Bone conduction testing delivers vibrations through the mastoid bone, skipping the outer and middle ear to specifically test the cochlea.[21]

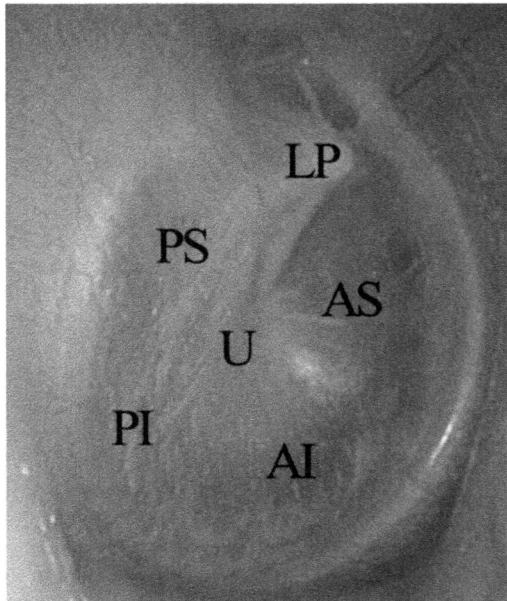

Fig. 2. Otoscopic examination of normal tympanic membrane. AI, anterior inferior quadrant; AS, anterior superior quadrant; LP, lateral process of the malleus; PI, posterior inferior quadrant; PS, posterior superior quadrant; U, umbo. (Beyea JA, Rohani SA, Ladak HM, Agrawal SK. Laser Doppler Vibrometry measurements of human cadaveric tympanic membrane vibration. Journal of Otolaryngology - Head & Neck Surgery. 2013;42(1). https://doi.org/10.1186/1916-0216-42-17)

If PTA is not readily available, other tests can be performed. The Automated Auditory Brainstem Response or Transient Evoked Otoacoustic Emissions (TEOAE) test measures inner ear hair cell vibrations after a stimulus like an electroencephalogram. It is easy to use and practical, but patients need to be sleeping or sedated. TEOAE does not assess defects proximal to the cochlea, so functional hearing loss or auditory neuropathies cannot be diagnosed. It is a good tool for people with learning disabilities, developmental delay, and speech or cognitive impairments as it is an objective form of measurement.

Automated hearing tests or boothless audiometry is an additional option, only requiring noise-canceling headphones. Digits-in-noise testing relies on speech recognition rather than pure tones. The WHO has created the "hearWHOpro" app for providers to use. There are also over 40 mobile apps to assess hearing, but none have been properly validated yet.[22]

Lastly, a proper neurologic assessment should be performed by PCPs. Defects in CNs V and VII can signify neuromas or stroke. CT or MRI is best done after audiology or ear, nose, throat (ENT) consultation given the low prevalence and diagnostic yield of advanced imaging and the risk that incidental findings may unnecessarily increase patient anxiety.[23]

TREATMENTS

For acute episodes of hearing loss with clear etiology found on history and examination, treating the underlying cause should be sufficient to restore normal hearing. Common

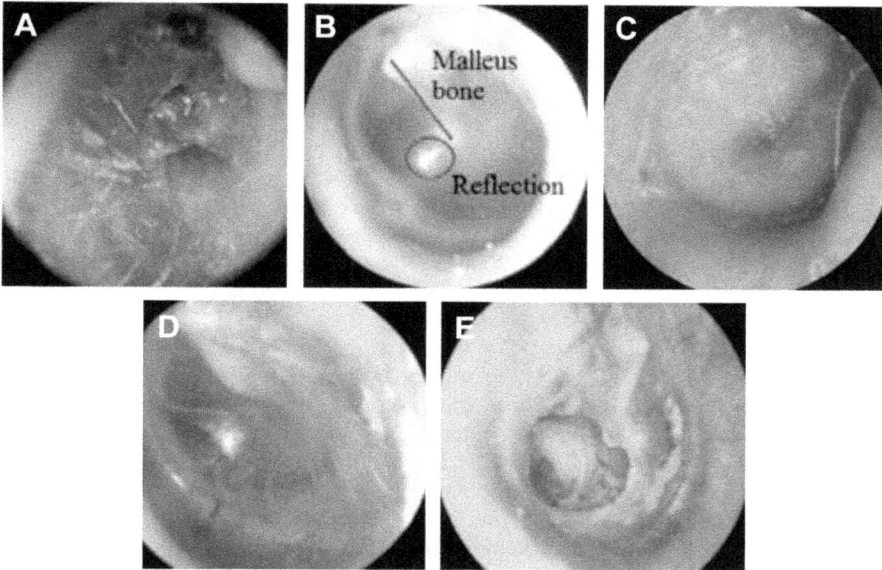

Fig. 3. (*A*) Obstructing wax in external ear canal obstructing visualization of TM; (*B*) normal TM; (*C*) acute otitis media (AOM) showing a bulging tympanic membrane (TM) with red color; (*D*) otitis media with effusion (OME) showing a retracted TM and fluid in the middle ear; and (*E*) chronic suppurative otitis media (CSOM) showing a TM perforation. (*With permission from Prof. Claude Laurent.*)

examples include removing cerumen with the use of irrigation, cerumenolytic liquids (none are superior to the others), or manual removal[24]; for otitis media, antibiotics can treat and prevent spread of infection, although there is equivocal evidence on the benefit of using antibiotics on long-term hearing outcomes.[25] Tympanostomy tubes can be considered for patients with recurrent ear infections.[26] Any ototoxic medications should be discontinued if appropriate.

Sudden onset hearing loss (<72 hours, >30 dB of loss) with no obvious etiology requires urgent audiological and ENT evaluation, and glucocorticoid treatment. PCPs play a crucial role in recognizing and facilitating the treatment of this audiological emergency.[27] Intratympanic steroids may have some benefit but also carry side effects such as pain, vertigo, persistent tympanic membrane perforation, tinnitus, infection, and tongue numbness. When used, steroids should be initiated within 2 weeks of hearing loss onset. When noise exposure is identified as the inciting cause for sudden onset hearing loss, N-acetylcysteine (NAC) therapy may have small benefit.[28–32] In 80% to 90% of cases, the etiology of sudden onset sensorineural hearing loss will not be found.

With chronic hearing impairment, consideration of the patient's age, hearing loss severity, socioeconomic context, communication needs and preferences, and the resources available are vital in forming the best plan to maximize function and quality of life. Mild-to-moderate hearing loss can be treated with hearing aids or personal sound amplification devices, while severe hearing loss can be treated with cochlear implants or alternative communication techniques (speech reaching and active listening training).

Hearing aids can improve quality of life even for the cognitively impaired, children, and individuals with severe hearing loss. Hearing aids cost anywhere from US$1000 to US$6000, with the average being US$2500.[33] Hearing aids can now be purchased over the counter but still require a medical examination to rule out red flag symptoms. An over the counter (OTC) hearing aid would not be a good choice for someone with severe loss, or hearing loss secondary to injury, illness, or underlying medical condition. However, they can be a cost-effective option when compared to traditional hearing aids as long as hearing recovery is greater than 55%.[34] Costs still remain high for the US public, whereas the wholesale cost for Veterans Affairs and the United Kingdom's national health service is US$300. Medicare will cover audiology treatments only if a licensed physician gives a referral, and while Medicare Advantage gives some hearing benefits, straight Medicare will not.[35]

Cochlear implants are Food and Drug Administration (FDA) approved for use in children with an intact cochlea and vestibulocochlear nerve. They must be aged 9 months and older, with hearing thresholds in the profound hearing loss range bilaterally. Recently, the FDA expanded the criteria to include children aged 24 months and older with severe bilateral hearing thresholds and children aged 5 years and older with single-sided deafness or asymmetric hearing thresholds with limited word recognition. Cochlear implants do not recreate normal hearing but help develop language and communication skills. Bone conduction and active middle ear implants are currently in development as an alternative.

Managing hearing loss is a multidisciplinary effort, involving auditory rehab, family-centered counseling, early intervention, speech language pathology, audiology, and school specialists who develop individual education plans. PCPs can counsel patients on adjusting their environment and communication techniques, such as reducing background noise, using face-to-face communication, rephrasing misheard statements, and summarizing heard statements to confirm comprehension.

PREVENTION

PCPs can prevent hearing loss with consistent and timely counseling. Sixty percent of acquired pediatric cases are avoidable, with over 19% attributed to not receiving routine vaccinations against rubella and meningitis. In the prenatal period, PCPs should emphasize adequate nutrition, properly washing hands and food, cooking to safe temperatures, and the role of breastfeeding in reducing otitis media.

For patients of all ages, reducing noise exposure to safer levels—especially in the electronics era—may be the most important "ear hygiene" practice clinicians can counsel patients on. Built-in decibel monitors or the Sound Level Meter App from the National Institute of Occupational Safety and Health are helpful tool for personal monitoring of noise exposure on smartphones. If these features are unavailable, a good rule of thumb is to reduce listening volume to 60% or less.

In noisy environments, use of earplugs, earmuffs, and canal caps should be advised, with formable foam earplugs an inexpensive and effective option. Patients should maintain distance from extremely loud noises and limit the time they are exposed to noise greater than 85 dB to no more than 8 hours per day. For reference, having to raise one's voice when speaking to someone 3 ft away may be a sign of environmental noise levels greater than 85 dB, a fact patients can be counseled on to prevent hearing loss.[36]

Educating patients can reduce noise exposure by 27.7%, with incremental cost-effectiveness ratios of US$10,657 per case counseled. Without intervention, the average cost for occupational noise-induced hearing loss per individual is US$64,172.[37,38]

Lastly, patients should be reminded that cotton tip applicators should only clean externally, to not insert objects or instill liquids in the ear unless directed by a clinician, and to avoid home remedies for the ears. If excessive earwax develops, patients may use peroxide as long as the ear canal is not dry or itching, as the peroxide may exacerbate this. Patients should maintain good nutrition and healthy lifestyle practices, avoid tobacco use, receive routine recommended immunizations, and seek prompt medical attention for ear pain, discharge, bleeding, or hearing loss[39] (**Fig. 4**).

DISCUSSION: CHALLENGES AND FUTURE DIRECTIONS

Almost all PCPs agree that hearing loss affects quality of life, but a large percentage of them are not routinely evaluating hearing impairment, citing lack of time, inadequate reimbursement, and uncertainties on whom and where to refer. Additionally, 48% of physicians in one survey reported not referring patients for further evaluation because they believed the hearing aids would be too expensive, or their patients would not live long enough to benefit.[38]

In reality, simple tests and even single-question screenings ("Do you have hearing problems?") are nearly as accurate as multiple-item questionnaires and handheld audiometers and can be easily incorporated into a clinic's workflow.[40]

PCPs should also recognize the role of social disadvantage on hearing loss. People living in poverty-stricken, refugee, immigrant, and rural communities may experience noise-filled, overcrowded housing and daycare, tobacco smoke, poor hygiene, and nutritional status. Hearing loss with these factors can then result in loss of educational potential or disability from work, and feed into generational cycles of poverty.[41,42] Patients from rural communities tend to be poorer and older, with significant distance, transportation, and financial barriers to being evaluated.[43] In these situations, PCPs should seek to reduce disparities by providing language

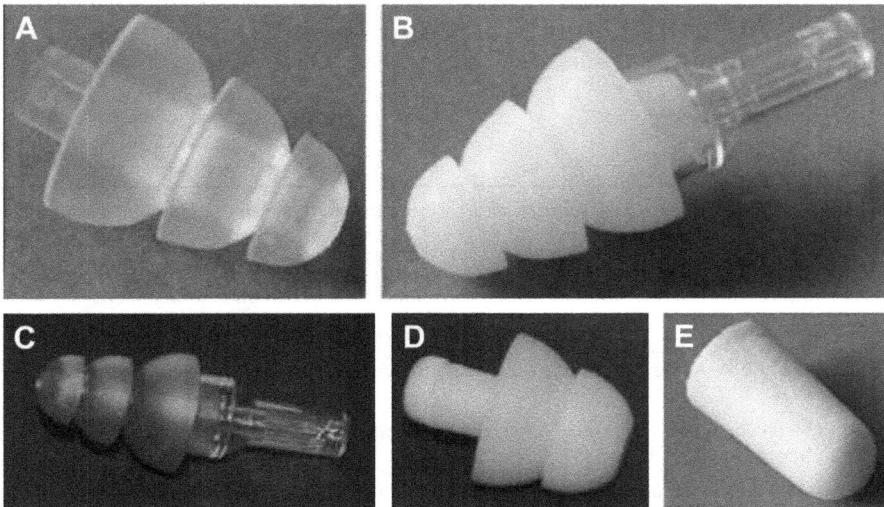

Fig. 4. Various sizes to conform to each individual ear canal size and shape. (*A*) Earplug 1 (11 mm; 4 mm); (*B*) Earplug 2 (13 mm; 16 mm); (*C*) Earplug 3 (9 mm; 16 mm); (*D*) Earplug 4 (11 mm; 8 mm); and (*E*) Earplug 5 (11 mm). (Bockstael, Annelies; Keppler, Hannah; Botteldooren, Dick. Musician earplugs: Appreciation and protection. Noise and Health 17(77):p 198-208, Jul–Aug 2015. https://doi.org/10.4103/1463-1741.160688.)

accommodations for hearing tests and consider Internet-based testing (where Internet access is available) or mobile health screenings since these can be comparable to PTA.[44]

PCPs should also accommodate people with hearing loss so they can properly access care. Using text-based and voice-phone-based scheduling can ensure appointments are made and avoid gaps in care. Investing in video remote interpretation when necessary would also ensure that a clinic does not discriminate against patients who use sign language.[45] With signing interpreters, clear language and avoiding medical jargon becomes essential as many medical terms lack signs.[46–48] Lastly, using validated tools designed for people with hearing loss to screen for other medical problems (eg, the Montreal Cognitive Assessment - Hearing Impairment [MOCA-H] for dementia[49]) and ensuring hearing is optimized through the use of hearing aids can help PCPs manage other chronic health problems better.[50]

With regards to hearing aids, obtaining one is only the first step. The lifespan of each averages 3 to 7 years and requires regular maintenance. About 18% to 38% of individuals with hearing aids experience interrupted use of them; 5.3% cease using them altogether. These patterns are associated with younger age, lower education, and lower income. Interrupted use was also associated with dementia and having a caregiver who helps with at least one activity of daily living. Managing complex medical needs may lead to minimizing the importance of hearing aid use. Clinicians should review treatment plans with caregivers—including hearing aid use—which may improve patient outcomes.[51]

SUMMARY

Hearing loss is a common disability that can affect individuals of any age. Many cases are preventable, and PCPs are perfectly situated to recognize, manage, and lead a multidisciplinary approach to hearing loss to maximize function and quality of life. Despite recent legislation approving OTC hearing aids, an enormous gap in the nation's hearing needs still remains. PCPs can address disparities by advocating for affordable devices, expanding insurance coverage, and appropriately compensating clinicians for managing an issue, which bears such individual and public health significance.

CLINICS CARE POINTS

- Hearing loss affects physical, mental, and socioeconomic health, particularly in the elderly (20% increase in mortality)

- The differential diagnosis is broad and often multifactorial; stratifying patients by age and taking an accurate history and examination can direct diagnosis and management

- Use a single question to screen for hearing loss ("Do you have difficulty with your hearing?")

- Aside from PTA, numerous tools are available to evaluate hearing loss even in primary care clinics

- Whispered voice test, finger rub, watch tick, and conversation are not accurate methods for evaluation

- Work in a multidisciplinary team; know the red flags for urgent ENT referral

- OTC hearing aids can be cost-effective for patients, but less effective in severe cases

- General counseling:
  o Keep volume on devices below 60%
  o Use hearing protection in noisy environments
  o Ear hygiene

- Make accommodations for patients who are hard of hearing to reduce barriers or gaps in care

DISCLOSURE

The authors have nothing to disclose.

REFERENCES

1. Humes LE. U.S. Population data on hearing loss, trouble hearing, and hearing-device use in adults: national health and nutrition examination survey, 2011-12, 2015-16, and 2017-20. Trends Hear 2023;27:23312165231160978. Available at: https://pubmed.ncbi.nlm.nih.gov/37016920/.
2. Genther DJ, Betz J, Pratt S, et al, Health ABC Study. Association of hearing impairment and mortality in older adults. J Gerontol A Biol Sci Med Sci 2015; 70(1):85–90. Available at: https://pubmed.ncbi.nlm.nih.gov/25024235/.
3. Lieu JEC, Kenna M, Anne S, et al. Hearing loss in children: a review. JAMA 2020; 324(21):2195–205. Available at: https://pubmed.ncbi.nlm.nih.gov/33258894/.
4. Michels TC, Duffy MT, Rogers DJ. Hearing loss in adults: differential diagnosis and treatment. Am Fam Physician 2019;100(2):98–108. PMID: 31305044.
5. World Health Organization. World report on hearing. World Health Organization; 2021. Available at: https://www.who.int/publications/i/item/9789240020481.
6. Sydlowski SA, Marinelli JP, Lohse CM, et al. Hearing health perceptions and literacy among primary healthcare providers in the United States: a national cross-sectional survey. Otol Neurotol 2022;43(8):894–9.
7. Feltner C, Wallace IF, Kistler CE, et al. Screening for hearing loss in older adults: an evidence review for the U.S. Preventive services task force. Rockville (MD): Agency for Healthcare Research and Quality (US); 2021.
8. Elzinga HBE, van Oorschot HD, Stegeman I, et al. Relation between otitis media and sensorineural hearing loss: a systematic review. BMJ Open 2021;11(8): e050108.
9. Lieu JEC, Kenna M, Anne S, et al. Hearing loss in children: a review. JAMA 2020; 324(21):2195–205.
10. Samocha-Bonet D, Wu B, Ryugo DK. Diabetes mellitus and hearing loss: a review. Ageing Res Rev 2021;71:101423. Epub 2021 Aug 9. Available at: https://pubmed.ncbi.nlm.nih.gov/34384902/.
11. Driscoll DP. OSHA technical manual (OTM) section III: chapter 5. OSHA. 2022. Available at: https://www.osha.gov/otm/section-3-health-hazards/chapter-5#affectedindustries.
12. Steyger PS. Mechanisms of ototoxicity and otoprotection. Otolaryngol Clin North Am 2021;54(6):1101–15. Available at: https://pubmed.ncbi.nlm.nih.gov/34774227/.
13. Hearing assessment in infants, children, and adolescents: recommendations beyond neonatal screening. Pediatrics 2023;152(3):e2023063288. Available at: https://pubmed.ncbi.nlm.nih.gov/37635686/.
14. Tuohimaa K, Loukusa S, Löppönen H, et al. Communication abilities in children with hearing loss - views of parents and daycare professionals. J Commun Disord 2022;99:106256.
15. Position statement: red flags-warning of ear disease. American Academy of Otolaryngology – Head and Neck Surgery 2021. Available at: https://www.entnet.org/resource/position-statement-red-flags-warning-of-ear-disease/.

16. McShea L, Giles K, Murphy A, et al. An alternative approach for detecting hearing loss in adults with learning disabilities. Br J Learn Disabil 2022;50(1):66–75.
17. Mankowski NL, Raggio BS. Otoscope exam. 2023 jan 16. In: StatPearls [internet]. Treasure Island (FL): StatPearls Publishing; 2023. Available at: https://www.ncbi.nlm.nih.gov/books/NBK553163/.
18. Wahid NWB, Hogan CJ, Attia M. Weber test. 2023 Jul 10. In: StatPearls [internet]. Treasure Island (FL): StatPearls Publishing; 2023. Available at: https://www.ncbi.nlm.nih.gov/books/NBK526135/.
19. Kong EL, Fowler JB. Rinne test. 2023 jan 30. In: StatPearls [internet]. Treasure Island (FL): StatPearls Publishing; 2024.
20. Pure-tone testing. American speech-language-hearing association. Available at: https://www.asha.org/public/hearing/pure-tone-testing/. Accessed February 16, 2024.
21. Irace AL, Sharma RK, Reed NS, et al. Smartphone-based applications to detect hearing loss: a review of current technology. J Am Geriatr Soc 2021;69(2):307–16.
22. Sajid IM, Frost K. Hear me out: rethinking internal auditory meatus magnetic resonance imaging in primary care. A cohort evaluation. J Laryngol Otol 2022;136(1):37–44.
23. Horton GA, Simpson MTW, Beyea MM, et al. Cerumen management: an updated clinical review and evidence-based approach for primary care physicians. J Prim Care Community Health 2020;11:2150132720904181. https://doi.org/10.1177/2150132720904181.
24. Mulvaney CA, Galbraith K, Webster KE, et al. Antibiotics for otitis media with effusion (OME) in children. Cochrane Database Syst Rev 2023;10:CD015254.
25. Rosenfeld RM, Tunkel DE, Schwartz SR, et al. Clinical practice guideline: tympanostomy tubes in children (update). Otolaryngol Head Neck Surg 2022;166(1_suppl):S1–55.
26. Prince ADP, Stucken EZ. Sudden sensorineural hearing loss: a diagnostic and therapeutic emergency. J Am Board Fam Med 2021;34(1):216–23.
27. Zhou Y, Zheng G, Zheng H, et al. Primary observation of early transtympanic steroid injection in patients with delayed treatment of noise-induced hearing loss. Audiol Neurootol 2013;18(2):89–94. Available at: https://pubmed.ncbi.nlm.nih.gov/23208457/.
28. Chang YS, Bang KH, Jeong B, et al. Effects of early intratympanic steroid injection in patients with acoustic trauma caused by gunshot noise. Acta Otolaryngol 2017;26:1–7. Available at: https://pubmed.ncbi.nlm.nih.gov/28125313/.
29. Plontke SK, Meisner C, Agrawal S, et al. Intratympanic corticosteroids for sudden sensorineural hearing loss. Cochrane Database Syst Rev 2022;7:CD008080 (English).
30. Jun Y, Mandrekar SJ. High-dose glucocorticoids for treating sudden hearing loss: cart before the horse? NEJM Evidence 2024;3(1):1–2.
31. Le TN, Straatman LV, Lea J, et al. Current insights in noise-induced hearing loss: a literature review of the underlying mechanism, pathophysiology, asymmetry, and management options. J Otolaryngol Head Neck Surg 2017;46(1):41. Available at: https://pubmed.ncbi.nlm.nih.gov/28535812/.
32. Rowden A, Iskander A, Dresden D, et al. Hearing aid cost and pricing: prescription and OTC options. Medical News Today; 2023. Available at: https://www.medicalnewstoday.com/articles/cost-of-hearing-aids.

33. Borre ED, Johri M, Dubno JR, et al. Potential clinical and economic outcomes of over-the-counter hearing aids in the US. JAMA Otolaryngol Head Neck Surg 2023;149(7):607–14.
34. National Institute on Deafness and Other Communication Disorders. Hearing protectors. NIH. Available at: https://www.nidcd.nih.gov/health/hearing-protectors. Accessed May 14, 2024.
35. Occupational Noise Exposure. Occupational safety and health administration website. Available at: https://www.osha.gov/noise. Accessed May 14, 2024.
36. Garcia SL, Smith KJ, Palmer C. Cost-effectiveness analysis of a military hearing conservation program. Mil Med 2018;183(9–10):e547–53. Available at: https://pubmed.ncbi.nlm.nih.gov/29425310/.
37. DeJonckheere M, McKee MM, Guetterman TC, et al. Implementation of a hearing loss screening intervention in primary care. Ann Fam Med 2021;19(5):388–95.
38. Berg S, Hunter JB, Jones SC. What doctors wish patients knew about proper ear care. AMA 2023. Available at: https://ama-assn.org/delivering-care/public-health/what-doctors-wish-patients-knew-about-proper-ear-care.
39. Tsimpida D, Kontopantelis E, Ashcroft DM, et al. Conceptual model of hearing health inequalities (HHI model): a critical interpretive synthesis. Trends Hear 2021;25. 23312165211002963.
40. Qian ZJ, Rehkopf DH. Association between social disadvantage and otitis media treatment in US children with commercial insurance. JAMA Otolaryngol Head Neck Surg 2022;149(1):7–14.
41. Ralli M, Marinelli A, De-Giorgio F, et al. Prevalence of otolaryngology diseases in an urban homeless population. Otolaryngol Head Neck Surg 2022;166(6):1022–7.
42. Barr M, Dally K, Duncan J. Service accessibility for children with hearing loss in rural areas of the United States and Canada. Int J Pediatr Otorhinolaryngol 2019;123:15–21.
43. Wang K, Wei W, Shi J, et al. Diagnostic accuracy of mobile health-based audiometry for the screening of hearing loss in adults: a systematic review and meta-analysis. Telemed J e Health 2023;29(10):1433–45.
44. Dawes P, Munro KJ, Frank TL, et al. Uptake of internet-delivered UK adult hearing assessment. Int J Audiol 2021;60(11):885–9.
45. Schniedewind E, Lindsay RP, Snow S. Comparison of access to primary care medical and dental appointments between simulated patients who were deaf and patients who could hear. JAMA Netw Open 2021;4(1):e2032207.
46. Lee PH, Spooner C, Harris MF. Access and communication for deaf individuals in Australian primary care. Health Expect 2021;24(6):1971–8.
47. de Oliveira P, Marciana P, Mendes da Silva G, et al. Access to primary healthcare services by people with disabilities. Andressa Suelly Rev Rene 2023;24(1):1–9.
48. Dawes P, Reeves D, Yeung WK, et al. Development and validation of the Montreal cognitive assessment for people with hearing impairment (MoCA-H). J Am Geriatr Soc 2023;71(5):1485–94.
49. Fioravante N, Deal JA, Willink A, et al. Preventive care utilization among adults with hearing loss in the United States. Semin Hear 2021;42(1):37–46.
50. Gahlon G, Garcia Morales EE, Assi L, et al. Factors associated with longitudinal patterns of hearing aid use. Innov Aging 2024;8(2):igae011.
51. Marcos-Alonso S, Almeida-Ayerve CN, Monopoli-Roca C, et al. Factors impacting the use or rejection of hearing aids-A systematic review and meta-analysis. J Clin Med 2023;12(12):4030.

Sinusitis

James Wilcox, MD, RMSK[a],*, Daniela Lobo, MD[b],
Sierra Anderson, MD[c,1]

KEYWORDS

- Sinusitis • Acute bacterial sinusitis • Chronic sinusitis • Rhinosinusitis
- Pott puffy tumor

KEY POINTS

- The most common etiology for sinusitis is a viral infection. Bacterial cases are associated with an antecedent viral upper respiratory tract infection with persistent symptoms lasting more than 10 days, worsening symptoms after initial improvement, or fever greater than 39 C (102.2 F).
- For patients with chronic sinusitis who have failed antibiotic trials and nasal saline irrigation, otolaryngology referral is recommended for evaluation with nasal endoscopy and consideration of surgical options such as adenoidectomy and endoscopic sinus surgery.
- Decongestants, antihistamines, and nasal irrigation are ineffective for children with acute bacterial sinusitis.

INTRODUCTION

Definitions

The paranasal sinuses are a group of 4 paired air-filled spaces: the maxillary, frontal, ethmoid, and sphenoidal sinuses, as demonstrated in **Fig. 1**. Sinusitis results from impaired mucociliary clearance and subsequent inflammation of the paranasal sinuses due to infection, allergies, or mechanical obstruction. In cases of rhinosinusitis, the inflammation extends to the nasal mucosa.

Types of sinusitis, depending on the duration, include

- *Acute infections*: up to 4 weeks
- *Subacute*: 4 to 12 weeks
- *Chronic*: lasts more than 12 weeks

[a] Department of Family Medicine, Indiana University School of Medicine, 980 Indiana Avenue Lockefield Village 1164, Indianapolis, IN 46202, USA; [b] Department of Family Medicine, Indiana University School of Medicine, 1040 Wishard Boulvard, Dunlap Building, Indianapolis, IN 46202, USA; [c] Department of Family Medicine, Indiana University School of Medicine, Indianapolis, IN, USA
[1] Present address: 2689 Maricopa Boulevard, Whitestown, IN 46075.
* Corresponding author.
E-mail address: jgwilcox@iu.edu

Prim Care Clin Office Pract 52 (2025) 87–97
https://doi.org/10.1016/j.pop.2024.09.010
primarycare.theclinics.com

SINUSITIS

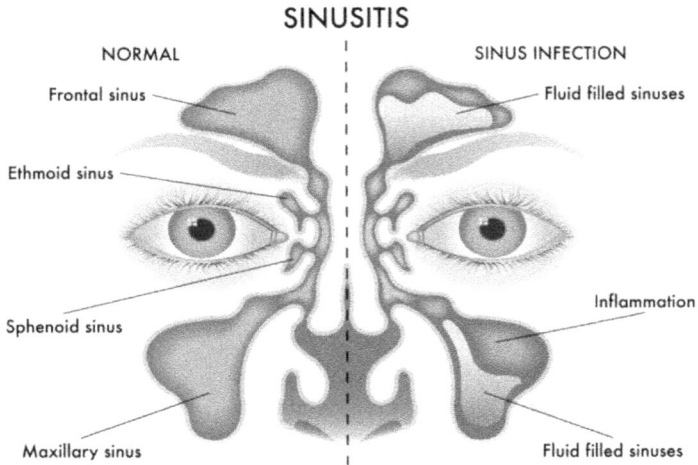

Fig. 1. Schematic cartoon of the sinuses and inflammation. (Rob9000/Shutterstock.com)

- *Recurrent infection*: involves 3 or more distinct episodes of sinusitis per year, with symptom-free intervals between episodes.

While the most common etiology is a viral infection, bacterial cases are associated with antecedent viral upper respiratory tract infections that have persistent symptoms lasting more than 10 days, worsening symptoms after initial improvement, or fever greater than 39 C (102.2 F).[1]

Epidemiology

In 2018, the Centers for Disease Control (CDC) reported 28.9 million adults diagnosed with sinusitis, resulting in 2.7 million visits to physician offices and 234,000 visits to emergency departments, with chronic sinusitis as the primary diagnosis.[2] In adults, the paranasal sinuses are a group of 4 paired air-filled spaces: the maxillary, frontal, ethmoid, and sphenoidal sinuses. In children, only the ethmoid and maxillary sinuses are present at birth.

Pathogenesis

Sinusitis results from impaired mucociliary clearance and subsequent inflammation of the paranasal sinuses due to infection, allergies, or mechanical obstruction. In cases of rhinosinusitis, the inflammation extends to the nasal mucosa. While viral causes like rhinovirus, influenza, and parainfluenza are the most common, bacterial causes are prominent as well. *Haemophilus influenzae, Streptococcus pneumoniae,* and *Moraxella catarrhalis* represent 60% to 70% of bacterial causes. Immunocompromised patients are susceptible to fungal infections caused by Aspergillus and Mucor species (for detailed infectious causes, see **Table 1**).

CLINICAL SIGNS AND SYMPTOMS

Sinusitis, characterized by inflammation of the paranasal sinuses, presents with a range of symptoms depending on the affected sinus and underlying cause. Common manifestations include facial pain, cough, congestion, postnasal drip, ear pain,

Table 1
Pathogens associated with sinusitis[3]

		Viruses	Bacteria
Adults	Most common	Rhino Influenza parainfluenza	*Streptococcus pneumoniae,* *Haemophilus influenzae,* *Moraxella catarrhalis,* *Streptococcus pyogenes,* *Staphylococcus aureus,* Other anaerobic bacteria
	Less common		*Fusobacterium nucleatum* *Prevotella and Porphyromonas* *Peptostreptococcus* species (spp)
Children	Most common	Rhino Influenza parainfluenza	*Streptococcus pneumoniae* *Haemophilus influenzae* *Moraxella catarrhalis*
	Less common		*Staphylococcus aureus* alpha-hemolytic streptococci

halitosis, hyposmia or anosmia, purulent nasal drainage, and nasal congestion or obstruction.[4]

- *Maxillary sinusitis:* This type of sinusitis is often associated with paranasal facial pain, retro-orbital discomfort, or maxillary dental pain. Patients may also experience purulent rhinorrhea and conjunctivitis, particularly in acute cases.[4]
- *Ethmoid sinusitis:* More prevalent in children, ethmoid sinusitis typically presents with periorbital pain and tenderness, often accompanied by nasal congestion and purulent discharge.[5]
- *Frontal sinusitis:* Patients with frontal sinus involvement commonly report a supraorbital headache, upper lid edema, and persistent rhinorrhea.[5]
- *Sphenoid sinusitis:* Although rare, sphenoid sinusitis can cause headaches and retro-orbital pain, often leading to diagnostic challenges due to its less frequent occurrence.[5]

In one study evaluating clinical diagnosis of sinusitis compared to computed tomography (CT), several symptoms had significant correlation seen on CT scan: preceding common cold, pain bending forward, purulent rhinorrhea, nasal voice, hyposmia or anosmia, unilateral frontal pain, double sickening, but only 2 signs correlated significantly: swollen nasal mucosa (98% sensitivity, 16% specificity) and purulent secretion (60% sensitivity, 89% specificity).[6]

DIAGNOSIS AND CRITERIA

The diagnosis of acute rhinosinusitis (ARS) in primary care is based on established clinical criteria. According to the 2015 otolaryngology guidelines,[7] ARS is suspected when patients present with up to 4 weeks of purulent nasal drainage (not clear) accompanied by nasal congestion andfacial pain, pressure, or fullness.

Distinguishing between viral and bacterial etiologies is crucial in management. Disease duration (>10 days) and worsening of symptoms before 10 days (double worsening sign) are key factors in this differentiation, guiding appropriate treatment strategies.[7] The "double worsening sign" is defined as acute sinusitis symptoms as above worsening within the first 10 days, rather than improving. Effectively their symptoms start off distressing, improve for a short time, then become worse again.

Pediatric Considerations

The ethmoid and maxillary sinuses are present at birth and are the most involved in sinusitis in children. Sphenoid sinuses form at the age of 3 to 5 years and begin to pneumatize at the age of 5 years but do not fully develop until the age of 20 to 30 years.[5] Frontal sinuses do not appear until the age of 7 to 8 years and remain incompletely pneumatized until late adolescence. Predisposing factors for acute bacterial sinusitis are diffuse mucositis secondary to viral rhinosinusitis in about 80% and allergic inflammation in about 20%. Less common predisposing factors include nonallergic rhinitis, cystic fibrosis, dysfunctional or insufficient immunoglobulins, ciliary dyskinesia, and anatomic abnormalities.[1]

PHYSICAL EXAMINATION

Diagnosis of rhinosinusitis is best supported by a thorough history and physical examination. Clinical findings that best rule in the diagnoses are purulent secretions in the middle meatus (positive likelihood ratio [LR+] 3.2) and the overall clinical impression of the clinician (LR+ 3.0), which impresses upon the clinician the role of experience and seeing many cases of sinusitis and other inflammatory and infectious diseases of the upper respiratory tract.[8] Four specific signs and symptoms have a high likelihood ratio and were independently associated with acute sinusitis: "double worsening sign," purulent rhinorrhea, purulent secretions, and erythrocyte sedimentation rate (ESR) greater than 10 had the highest likelihood ratios associated with acute sinusitis. A combination of at least 3 of these 4 symptoms and signs gave a specificity of 81% and a sensitivity of 66%.[6] The clinical findings that best rule out rhinosinusitis are the overall clinical impression (LR −0.37), normal transillumination (LR 0.55), the absence of preceding respiratory tract infection (LR− 0.48), any nasal discharge (LR− 0.49), and lack of purulent nasal discharge (LR −0.54).[8]

DIAGNOSTIC TESTS

While diagnostic testing is often not needed after a clinical diagnosis of sinusitis, one study found the prevalence of bacterial growth on cultures from patients clinically diagnosed with sinusitis was only about 52.5% to 61.1% (Smith 34) that demonstrates that clinical evaluation may overdiagnose bacterial sinusitis about half of the time. When diagnostic accuracy is essential, several tests have been studied (see **Table 2** for a detailed list of diagnostic test likelihood).

Radiograph and ultrasound are both relatively quick imaging modalities used to evaluate sinus infection. Radiographs have been utilized for decades to evaluate sinus inflammation and disease. One study compared radiograph to a reference standard of nasal aspiration using sinus opacity or fluid as the criterion for sinusitis; radiography had sensitivity of 73% and specificity of 80%. Studies evaluating ultrasonography revealed substantial variation in test performance.[9] While one small study[10] of 41 patients in 1992 compared ultrasound to a CT standard found that sensitivities for ultrasound of the maxillary, frontal, and ethmoid sinuses were 100% and specificity 94% to 100%, this high accuracy has not been reproduced. One more recent study[11] compared ultrasound to surgical outcomes and found that the sensitivity was significantly lower regarding the maxillary sinus (88%), the ethmoid sinus (53%), and the frontal sinus (45%).

CT, as seen in **Fig. 2**, has been the diagnostic test of choice to diagnose and evaluate disease severity in chronic rhinosinusitis (CRS), and more specifically to aid in surgical planning. The American College of Radiography Appropriateness Criteria

Table 2
Diagnostic tests for sinusitis

Test	+Likelihood Ratio	-Likelihood Ratio
Sedimentation Rate[17]	(>30) LR+ 4.08 (>40) LR+ 7.40	(<10) LR− 0.57
C-reactive Protein[17]	(>20) LR+ 2.92	(<10) LR− 0.45
Direct Nasal Endoscopy[16]	LR+ 3.1	LR− 0.36
Anterior Rhinoscopy[4]	LR+ 3.2, LR+ 5.3, or LR+ 11.0 (depending on location of discharge)	LR− 0.2
CT[11]	LR+ 2.9	LR− 0.04
Radiograph[9]	LR+ 3.6	LR− 0.34
Ultrasound[11]	LR+ 3.6	LR− 0.15

update on Sinonasal Disease in 2021 recommends first using CT of maxillofacial without intravenous (IV) contrast for acute recurrent sinusitis or CRS, or with contrast if there is a suspected complication, like orbital complications or adjacent intracranial complications. CT enables better surgical planning than ultrasound or radiograph given its detailed depiction of sinonasal anatomy and can be used for surgical image-guidance systems.[12] Although CT scan has been the gold standard for diagnosis for decades now, it is still not a perfect test. One dual cohort study found the sensitivity and specificity of CT with Lund criteria to be 85% and 59%, respectively.[13] The Lund-Mackay scoring system is a standardized method used to evaluate the severity of CRS CT scans. It assesses 6 sinus regions on each side of the face, including the maxillary, ethmoid, sphenoid, and frontal sinuses, as well as the ostiomeatal complex. Each region is scored from 0 to 2, with 0 indicating no abnormality, 1 indicating partial opacification (blockage or fluid), and 2 indicating complete opacification. The total score reflects the overall severity of sinus disease. The Lund-Mackay scoring system is useful for quantifying the extent of CRS but has limitations in specificity, meaning it may sometimes indicate sinus disease when it is not present.

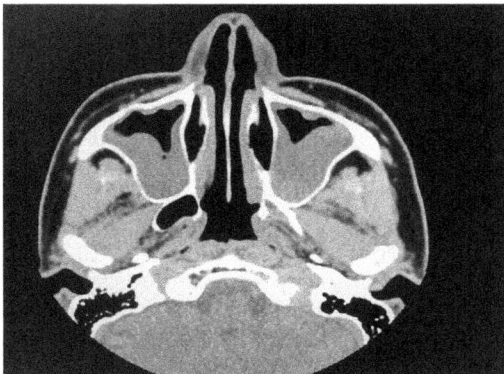

Fig. 2. CT scan of sinusitis with air fluid levels, inflammation, and purulent fluid in the maxillary sinuses. (Karan Bunjean/Shutterstock.com)

One study demonstrated this when the investigators found no correlation of CT findings with areas responsible for facial pain or pressure in patients.[14] Although CT is the most widely used, MRI might be an effective alternative when needing repeat tests or follow-up imaging. One study found that when using Lund-Mackay system scores in conjunction with CT, the likelihood of true sinus disease from CT-based and MRI-based scoring agreed in 85.4% of the cases evaluated.[15] The American College of Radiography Appropriateness Criteria lists MRI of the orbits, face, and neck without and with IV contrast as either "appropriate" or "may be appropriate" for each of the sinusitis concerns listed earlier. Additionally, it was noted that MRI might provide better information for certain conditions like soft tissue masses or cancers than CT with contrast did.

Direct nasal endoscopy showed a high correlation (r = .8543) between endoscopy and CT in terms of the diagnostic accuracy for CRS. The sensitivity and specificity were fair at 72.6% and 76.7%, respectively.[16] Laboratory evaluation can be performed at the bedside to aid in diagnosis of acute sinusitis. There is moderate evidence that an ESR of less than 10 for negative or greater than 30 for positive provides a sensitivity of 50% and specificity of 88%. If a cutoff of 40 is used, the specificity increases to 93%. Similarly, C-reactive protein (CRP) is another possible indicator of infection. A CRP level less than 10 mg/L for negative and greater than 20 for positive resulted in a sensitivity of 65% and a specificity of 78%.[17]

Complications

Severe complications from sphenoid sinusitis include cranial neuropathies, cavernous sinus thrombosis, meningitis, and intracranial abscess.[18,19] Proptosis or impairment of extraocular muscle movement suggests periorbital and orbital cellulitis, usually from the extension of an ethmoidal infection.

Predisposing factors for acute bacterial sinusitis are diffuse mucositis secondary to viral rhinosinusitis in about 80% and allergic inflammation in about 20%. Less common predisposing factors include nonallergic rhinitis, cystic fibrosis, dysfunctional or insufficient immunoglobulins, ciliary dyskinesia, and anatomic abnormalities.[1]

Pott's puffy tumor is a rare complication of a sinusitis infection by direct extension to the skull, resulting in osteomyelitis and subperiosteal abscess formation, clinically presenting as a boggy, tender swelling overlying the forehead. It is most commonly seen in pediatrics and young adolescents due to the pneumatization process and venous drainage, but it can also be diagnosed in adults.

MEDICAL MANAGEMENT

The mainstay of treatment of viral infections is supportive care, typically resolving within 10 days using self-care modalities such as humidification therapies, nasal washes, over-the-counter decongestants, anti-cough medicines, and rest with hydration.[20,21] If symptomatology is not improving overtime but worsening, it is appropriate to start more aggressive treatment with antibiotics.[22]

Prolonged infections are empirically treated with Amoxicillin 500 mg TID/875 mg twice daily (BID) or Amoxicillin with clavulanic acid 500/125 mg three times daily (TID) or 875/125 mg BID. For pediatrics, standard dosing is 45 mg/kg/day BID for both. High dosing is reserved for patients who are not responding to standard dosing or populations endemic to acute bacterial rhinosinusitis (ABRS), which is 80 to 90 mg/kg/day. Treatment should continue for 5 to 7 days in adults and 10 to 14 days in children.[3] Switching to broad-spectrum antibiotics may also be appropriate if symptoms have not improved by 7 days. It may be necessary to perform further evaluation to identify the cause of infection through laboratory testing, cultures, and other more invasive procedures. Additional microbial coverage with metronidazole or clindamycin is recommended if patients are still disease burdened.[3,23]

Children with uncomplicated rhinosinusitis should be allowed up to 10 days of symptomatic treatment. Those who are symptomatic for longer periods of time raise concern about bacterial causes of infection. In these cases, initiating oral antibiotics is suggested. Evidenced in the American Academy of Pediatrics guidelines, the first-line treatment is amoxicillin that can be given with or without clavulanate.[24] Though there is no great evidence for which antibiotics to choose in pediatric rhinosinusitis, but based on evaluation of defining data, any penicillin agent is the recommended first-line treatment.[25] For patients with penicillin allergy are unresponsive to initial amoxicillin treatment, they can be treated safely with cephalosporins like cefdinir, cefuroxime, or cefpodoxime.[24]

For patients with chronic sinusitis, treatment should be aimed toward covering the most common pathogen, S pneumoniae, and have efficacy for higher incidence beta-lactamase-producing organisms that are more common in chronic infections.[3]

Most cases can be treated as outpatient; however, hospitalization with IV antibiotics may be required in more severe cases of sinusitis affecting the sphenoid sinuses, causing air-fluid levels, or in immunocompromised patients. Sinusitis caused by fungal infections has a much higher morbidity and mortality and should be addressed immediately and aggressively in a hospital setting.[26]

Recurrence/Chronic Sinusitis

CRS is defined by the presence of at least 2 out of 4 cardinal symptoms: facial pain/pressure, hyposmia/anosmia, nasal drainage, and nasal obstruction, with symptoms lasting more than 12 weeks and it may occur with or without nasal polyps.[27]

Indications for Surgical Referral

Endoscopic sinus surgery may be effective when medical management fails. Paranasal sinuses are a complex labyrinth of cells that drain into the nose. An essential feature of sinus health is the patency of the sinus openings to allow ventilation and drainage. Equally important is the status of the mucosa and cilia. Surgery usually addresses the patency issue but not the mucosa or the cilia. Modern-day sinus surgery attempts to open and ventilate the sinuses with as minimal collateral damage to adjacent mucosa as possible.[28] Studies have shown that combined balloon Eustachian tuboplasty and functional endoscopic sinus surgery (FESS) could decrease otologic symptoms and improve Eustachian tube function.[29,30] These procedures are used in more severe cases of ARS, recurrent rhinosinusitis, or CRS who have failed medical management.[20,23] In some instances, it may be appropriate to continue medical management after surgical intervention.

Children who have asthma, gastroesophageal reflux disease, or other chronic respiratory diseases such as cystic fibrosis are more prone to requiring surgical intervention for ARS/CRS.[31]

EMERGING THERAPIES/EMERGING TREATMENT

In 2021, a meta-analysis showed primary outcomes on disease-specific health-related quality of life (HRQL), disease severity, and serious adverse events. Monoclonal antibodies are biologic products already evaluated in other inflammatory conditions (eg, asthma and atopic dermatitis). Almost all participants in the included studies had nasal polyps (99.8%) and used topical nasal steroids for their CRS symptoms. In these patients, dupilumab improved disease-specific HRQL compared to placebo. It may also result in a reduction in disease severity and a decrease in the number of serious adverse events. Therapeutic ultrasound is becoming an emerging possible technique for CRS. A systematic review in 2021 found 9 studies with significant improvement in symptoms and relief of the pathology. However, the studies were small, of short duration, and a high risk of bias per the authors.[32]

DISCUSSION

Sinusitis is a prevalent medical condition characterized by inflammation of the paranasal sinuses, often triggered by viral, bacterial, or fungal infections. Sinusitis affects millions worldwide, about 28.9 million people are affected in the United States each year,[33] significantly impacting quality of life and health care costs. Understanding the underlying pathophysiology is crucial, as sinusitis can be acute, subacute, recurrent acute, or chronic, each presenting with distinct clinical features and treatment approaches.

Clinically, diagnosis relies on a combination of clinical evaluation, imaging studies, and, occasionally, nasal endoscopy. Recent advances in imaging techniques, such as CT and MRI, have enhanced diagnostic accuracy. Management strategies encompass both pharmacologic and non-pharmacological interventions. Corticosteroids and nasal saline irrigation effectively reduce inflammation and promote sinus drainage, whereas antibiotics are commonly prescribed for bacterial sinusitis. Treatment of recurrent sinusitis can pose significant challenges. Surgical interventions, including FESS, may be warranted in chronic or recurrent sinusitis resistant to medical therapy. Recent advancements in sinusitis treatment, such as biologics targeting specific inflammatory pathways, may improve patient outcomes and decrease disease burden.

Sinusitis remains a prevalent and challenging condition, necessitating a multifaceted approach to diagnosis and management. Continued research efforts are crucial to elucidate the underlying mechanisms of sinusitis further and develop innovative therapeutic strategies to improve patient outcomes and quality of life.

SUMMARY

In conclusion, sinusitis is a prevalent inflammatory condition affecting the paranasal sinuses, with diverse etiologies including viral, bacterial, and fungal infections. Sinusitis, an inflammation of the paranasal sinuses, varies in presentation from acute to chronic forms, with each type requiring different therapeutic approaches. Diagnosis typically involves clinical evaluation, while sometimes imaging studies and nasal endoscopy can help with diagnosis and surgical planning. Management includes pharmacologic treatments like intranasal corticosteroids for reducing inflammation, and sometimes antibiotics when bacterial infection is suspected, alongside non-pharmacological measures such as nasal saline irrigation. In refractory cases, surgical interventions such as FESS are considered. Emerging treatments, including biologics and minimally invasive procedures, show promise as alternative management options.

CLINICS CARE POINTS

- Chronic sinusitis may be due to mucoid retention cysts, deviated septum, or nasal polyps. Refer to otolaryngology (ENT) for possible surgery.[18]

- For patients with chronic sinusitis who have failed antibiotic trials and nasal saline irrigation, an ENT referral is recommended for evaluation with nasal endoscopy and consideration of surgical options such as adenoidectomy and FESS.[1]
- Consider fungal etiologies in immunocompromised patients such as those with uncontrolled diabetes mellitus, human immunodeficiency virus positive, patients undergoing active cancer treatment, and patients on immunosuppressants for an organ transplant or rheumatologic conditions.
- Children with recurrent or refractory sinusitis should be evaluated for immune deficiencies or consider comorbid illnesses such as cystic fibrosis.[1,18]
- Decongestants, antihistamines, and nasal irrigation are ineffective for children with acute bacterial sinusitis.[34]

DECLARATION OF ARTIFICAL INTELLIGENCE (AI) AND AI-ASSISTED TECHNOLOGIES IN THE WRITING PROCESS

During the preparation of this work the author(s) used ChatGPT v3.5 to help with phrasing of sentences for publication and organization of references. After using this tool/service, the author(s) reviewed and edited the content as needed and take(s) full responsibility for the content of the publication.

DISCLOSURE

The authors have no financial responsibilities to disclose.

REFERENCES

1. Cohen JS, Agrawal D. Nose and sinus disorders in infants and children. In: Tintinalli JE, Ma O, Yealy DM, et al, editors. Tintinalli's emergency medicine: a comprehensive study guide. 9th edition. McGraw-Hill Education; 2020. Available at: https://accessmedicine-mhmedical-com.proxy.ulib.uits.iu.edu/content.aspx?bookid=2353&sectionid=189593704. Accessed February 28, 2024.
2. Santo L. and Okeyode T., National ambulatory medical care survey: 2018 national summary tables, Available at: https://www.cdc.gov/nchs/data/ahcd/namcs_summary/2018-namcs-web-tables-508.pdf (Accessed 17 April 2024).
3. Brook I. Microbiology of chronic rhinosinusitis. Eur J Clin Microbiol Infect Dis 2016;35:1059–68.
4. Autio TJ, Koskenkorva T, Närkiö M, et al. Diagnostic accuracy of history and physical examination in bacterial acute rhinosinusitis. Laryngoscope 2015; 125(7):1541–6.
5. DeBoer DL, Kwon E. Acute sinusitis. In: StatPearls [internet]. Treasure Island (FL): StatPearls Publishing; 2024. Available at: https://www.ncbi.nlm.nih.gov/books/NBK547701/.
6. Lindbaek M, Hjortdahl P, Johnsen UL. Use of symptoms, signs, and blood tests to diagnose acute sinus infections in primary care: comparison with computed tomography. Fam Med 1996;28(3):183–8.
7. Rosenfeld RM, Piccirillo JF, Chandrasekhar SS, et al. Clinical practice guideline (update): adult sinusitis. Otolaryngol Head Neck Surg 2015;152(2 Suppl). https://doi.org/10.1177/0194599815572097.
8. Ebell MH, McKay B, Dale A, et al. Accuracy of signs and symptoms for the diagnosis of acute rhinosinusitis and acute bacterial rhinosinusitis. Ann Fam Med 2019;17(2):164–72.

9. Engels EA, Terrin N, Barza M, et al. Meta-analysis of diagnostic tests for acute sinusitis. J Clin Epidemiol 2000;53(8):852–62.

10. Gianoli GJ, Mann WJ, Miller RH. B-mode ultrasonography of the paranasal sinuses compared with CT findings. Otolaryngol Head Neck Surg 1992;107(6 Pt 1):713–20.

11. Bozzato A, Arens C, Linxweiler M, et al. Multicenter observational study to evaluate the diagnostic value of sonography in patients with chronic rhinosinusitis. Diagnostics 2022;12(9):2065.

12. Hagiwara M, Policeni B, Juliano AF, et al, Expert Panel on Neurological Imaging. ACR appropriateness Criteria® sinonasal disease: 2021 update. J Am Coll Radiol 2022;19(5S). https://doi.org/10.1016/j.jacr.2022.02.011.

13. Bhattacharyya N, Fried MP. The accuracy of computed tomography in the diagnosis of chronic rhinosinusitis. Laryngoscope 2003;113(1):125–9.

14. Holbrook EH, Brown CL, Lyden ER, et al. Lack of significant correlation between rhinosinusitis symptoms and specific regions of sinus computer tomography scans. Am J Rhinol 2005;19(4):382–7.

15. Lin HW, Bhattacharyya N. Diagnostic and staging accuracy of magnetic resonance imaging for the assessment of sinonasal disease. Am J Rhinol Allergy 2009;23(1):36–9.

16. Kim DH, Seo Y, Kim KM, et al. Usefulness of nasal endoscopy for diagnosing patients with chronic rhinosinusitis: a meta-analysis. Am J Rhinol Allergy 2020;34(2):306–14.

17. Ebell MH, McKay B, Guilbault R, et al. Diagnosis of acute rhinosinusitis in primary care: a systematic review of test accuracy. Br J Gen Pract 2016;66(650) https://doi.org/10.3399/bjgp16X686581.

18. Jauch EC, Hall G, Knoop KJ. Acute sinusitis. In: Knoop KJ, Stack LB, Storrow AB, et al, editors. The atlas of emergency medicine. 5th edition. McGraw-Hill; 2021. Available at: https://accessmedicine-mhmedical-com.proxy.ulib.uits.iu.edu/content.aspx?bookid=2969&sectionid=250456275. Accessed February 28, 2024.

19. Sadineni RT, Velicheti S, Kondragunta CS, et al. Multiple cerebrovascular complications due to sphenoid sinusitis. J Clin Diagn Res 2016;10(11). https://doi.org/10.7860/JCDR/2016/23899.8905.

20. Zalmanovici Trestioreanu A, Barua A, Pertzov B. Cyclamen europaeum extract for acute sinusitis. Cochrane Database Syst Rev 2018;5. https://doi.org/10.1002/14651858.CD011341.pub2.

21. DeBoer DL, Kwon E. Acute sinusitis. 2023 aug 7. In: StatPearls [internet]. Treasure Island (FL): StatPearls Publishing; 2024.

22. Wyler B, Mallon WK. Sinusitis update. Emerg Med Clin North Am 2019;37(1):41–54.

23. Isaacson G. Surgical treatment of pediatric rhinosinusitis. Minerva Pediatr 2015;67(4):357–68.

24. Wald ER, Applegate KE, Bordley C, et al. Clinical practice guideline for the diagnosis and management of acute bacterial sinusitis in children aged 1 to 18 years. Pediatrics 2013;132(1):e262–80.

25. Ramadan HH, Chaiban R, Makary C. Pediatric rhinosinusitis. Pediatr Clin North Am 2022;69(2):275–86.

26. Mancuso RF. Pediatric allergic fungal sinusitis: a clinical review. Pediatr Ann 2021;50(7). https://doi.org/10.3928/19382359-20210706-01.

27. Sedaghat AR. Chronic rhinosinusitis. Am Fam Physician 2017;96(8):500–6.

28. Witterick IJ, Kolenda J. Surgical management of chronic rhinosinusitis. Immunol Allergy Clin North Am 2004;24(1):119–34.

29. Hsieh CY, Lin WC, Lin CC, et al. Combined balloon Eustachian tuboplasty/endo-scopic sinus surgery for patients with chronic rhinosinusitis and Eustachian tube dysfunction. Int Forum Allergy Rhinol 2024. https://doi.org/10.1002/alr.23341.
30. Chen X, Dang H, Chen Q, et al. Endoscopic sinus surgery improves Eustachian tube function in patients with chronic rhinosinusitis: a multicenter prospective study. Rhinology 2021;59(6):560–6.
31. Levine CG, Casiano RR. Revision functional endoscopic sinus surgery. Otolar-yngol Clin North Am 2017;50(1):143–64.
32. Da Silva GS, Dos Santos Isoppo K. Therapeutic ultrasound as a treatment for chronic rhinosinusitis: a systematic review. Clin Respir J 2021;15(12):1275–85.
33. Centers for Disease Control and Prevention. Summary health statistics: national health interview survey. Hyattsville, MD: National Center for Health Statistics; 2018. Available at: https://www.cdc.gov/nchs/fastats/sinuses.htm.
34. Shaikh N, Wald ER, Pi M. Decongestants, antihistamines and nasal irrigation for acute sinusitis in children. Cochrane Database Syst Rev 2012;9. https://doi.org/10.1002/14651858.CD007909.pub3.

Pharyngitis

Allison Holley, MD*, Sarah Wiggill, MD, MSc

KEYWORDS

- Pharyngitis • Strep throat • Antibiotic stewardship • Centor criteria
- Rheumatic fever • Group a streptococcal • Tonsillectomy • Acid reflux

KEY POINTS

- Etiologies of pharyngitis include viral, bacterial, fungal organisms, trauma, medication side effects, allergens, and irritants.
- Serious and life-threatening complications can develop when bacterial (especially group A streptococcus) pharyngitis infections are not appropriately and promptly treated; however, misdiagnosis of other infectious and noninfectious causes of pharyngitis also results in potentially serious complications.
- Thorough history-taking and skilled physical examination along with the utilization of clinical decision tools such as Centor criteria, McIsaac, and Fever-PAIN coupled with appropriate testing can help clinicians ascertain the appropriate treatment and avoid prescribing unnecessary antibiotics that can lead to adverse events and antibiotic resistance.
- Recurrent or persistent cases of pharyngitis are most commonly caused by treatment regimen nonadherence or misdiagnosis.

INTRODUCTION

Pharyngitis is a common diagnosis in the primary care office making up an estimated 24 million cases per year in the United States.[1] Pharyngitis is defined as inflammation of the pharynx and adjacent tissues, and the most common etiologies include viral, bacterial, or fungal origin.[2] Less common causes of pharyngitis include trauma, medication side effects, allergies, and irritants.[3] Even though the single most common cause of pharyngitis is viral with approximately 50% to 80% of cases,[4] and group A streptococcal pharyngitis makes up only about 10% of cases, more than 60% of patients are treated with antibiotics.[1] Utilizing clinical decision tools, ensuring appropriate testing, and following current guidelines can help clinicians ascertain the appropriate treatment and avoid prescribing unnecessary antibiotics that can lead to adverse events and antibiotic resistance.

Department of Family Medicine, Florida Atlantic University College of Medicine, Boca Raton, FL, USA
* Corresponding author. 777 Glades Road BC-71, Boca Raton, FL 33431.
E-mail address: holleya@health.fau.edu

Prim Care Clin Office Pract 52 (2025) 99–109
https://doi.org/10.1016/j.pop.2024.09.011   **primarycare.theclinics.com**

ETIOLOGY

The main 2 categories of pharyngitis etiology are infectious and noninfectious causes. Infectious causes of pharyngitis include viral, bacterial, and fungal causes. Noninfectious causes include trauma such as intubation, accidents, voice strain, irritants such as chemicals, pollutants, smoking or inhalation injury, environmental allergens, stomach acid (as seen in laryngopharyngeal reflux [LPR]), dry or cold air, and medication side effect.[3]

Infectious Causes

Viral pathogens

The majority of infectious pharyngitis cases is due to viral pathogens. The leading viral causes of pharyngitis include rhinovirus, adenovirus, and coronavirus (including coronavirus disease 2019 [COVID-19]). Influenza, parainfluenza, and respiratory syncytial virus are other common viral causes. Less common viral causes include human immunodeficiency virus (HIV), herpes, Epstein-Barr, cytomegalovirus, and coxsackie viruses.[2,4,5]

Bacterial pathogens

Group A streptococcus (GAS) is thought to be the most common bacterial pathogen responsible for pharyngitis making up approximately 5% to 15% of cases in adults and 20% to 30% of cases in children.[5] Group C and G streptococcus, *Arcanobacterium haemolyticum*, *Fusobacterium necrophorum*, *Mycoplasma pneumoniae*, *Chlamydia pneumoniae*, and *Corynebacterium diphtheriae* are other bacterial causes.[5,6] Some of these less common bacterial causes are more likely to be found in certain patient populations. For example, Group C and G streptococcus and *F necrophorum* are more likely to be found in outbreaks on college campuses and in student health clinics.[6] Other pathogens such as *C diphtheriae* are more likely to be found in underdeveloped countries where lack of access to care and low vaccination rates contribute to higher prevalence.[7] High-risk sexual behavior may place patients at risk for rare causes of bacterial pharyngitis from sexually transmitted infections such as *Treponema pallidum* and *Neisseria gonorrhoeae* as well as from viruses such as HIV.[2,4,8]

Fungal pathogens

Candida albicans is the main fungal pathogen that can cause pharyngitis, but it is mainly seen in the immunocompromised patient population or those using inhaled corticosteroids.[3]

Noninfectious Causes

Noninfectious causes are a diagnosis of exclusion and are not well-studied. A detailed history will aid clinicians in appropriately identifying these causes of pharyngitis.[3]

Trauma

Use of laryngeal mask airways or tracheal intubation increases the risk of trauma-induced pharyngitis. In patients undergoing intubation, a range of 28% to 70% report sore throat, and about 3% to 21% report sore throat after laryngeal mask airway use.[3] Snoring, yelling, and frequent talking can also lead to sore throat.

Irritants

Smokers and patients exposed to second-hand smoke may also develop symptoms of pharyngitis.[3] Increased use of electronic cigarettes and inhaled marijuana, especially among adolescents and young adults, has resulted in increased incidence of irritant-induced pharyngitis.[9,10] Air pollution most commonly seen in large cities and due to frequent exposure to traffic fumes can cause sore throat. Industrial particulates such as seen with woodworking, cement working, or exhaust fumes from industrial machines as well as chemicals such as boron acid, volatile organic compounds, and oil spills also contribute to work-related injuries. Indoor air pollution, often termed "sick building syndrome," can cause irritant-induced pharyngitis along with a myriad of other complaints that are generally caused by faulty air cooling/heating/ventilation systems or mold. Cold temperature and low humidity are also factors that can lead to pharyngitis.[3]

Laryngopharyngeal reflux
LPR is a common cause of pharyngeal irritation. It is difficult to diagnose due to unreliable findings on laryngoscopy and pH monitoring but often responds well to a trial of proton pump inhibitors (PPIs).[11]

Medications
The most common medications that may cause throat pain usually occur as a result of pill esophagitis, which can cause inflammation of the esophagus and surrounding tissues including the pharynx. Antibiotics (most notably doxycycline), nonsteroidal anti-inflammatory drugs (NSAIDs), and bisphosphonates are the most common medications involved, but often the likelihood of this adverse effect occurring can be mitigated by having patients take these medications while seated upright, with a large glass of water, and not to recline or lie down directly after taking the medications.[12] Angiotensin-converting enzyme-inhibitors and chemotherapy are other medications that may also contribute to symptoms of sore throat.[3]

CLINICAL PRESENTATION

The primary presenting symptom of pharyngitis, regardless of etiology, is sore throat. Other presenting symptoms and signs of pharyngitis may vary by pathogen and cause. Group A streptococcal pharyngitis generally presents with tonsillar exudate, fever, and/or tender anterior chain lymphadenopathy. It is extremely rare in children aged under 3 years. Viral pharyngitis is more likely to be accompanied by cough and nasal congestion.[1] Epstein-Barr virus (EBV) and cytomegalovirus (CMV) are 2 viral pathogens that can cause infectious mononucleosis, which is recognized by a triad of symptoms including fever, pharyngitis, and lymphadenopathy.[13,14] Candidiasis is more likely to present with white or erythematous patches in the mouth and throat and is more common in the immunocompromised host although can also be present in immunocompetent hosts.[15] LPR usually presents with pharyngeal erythema and may be accompanied by hoarseness, sore throat, throat clearing, globus sensation, and cough.[11]

EVALUATION
Clinical Decision Tools

Clinical decision tools that have been substantiated specifically for streptococcal pharyngitis include Centor, McIsaac (which is also known as Modified Centor), and Fever-PAIN, which are all equivocal. When coupled with appropriate rapid testing, they can help decrease inappropriate antibiotic use.[1,16]

Centor criteria give 1 point for each of the following: lack of cough, tonsillar exudate or swelling, fever (temperature $\geq 100.4°F$), swollen, tender anterior cervical chain lymphadenopathy.

McIsaac (modified Centor) gives 1 point to each of those listed in Centor, but also adds age as a factor by affording an additional 1 point to those patients aged 3 to

14 years, 0 points for those aged 15 to 44 years, and −1 (subtract 1 point) for those aged 45 years and older.

Fever-PAIN gives 1 point for each of the following: absence of cough or coryza, feverishness in the last 24 hours, intensely inflamed tonsils, purulent tonsils, presentation within 3 days of symptom onset.

Each of these clinical decision tools uses the same risk scoring with a score of 0 to 1 being considered low risk, 2 to 3 intermediate risk, and 4 to 5 high risk. Patients who are at low risk should not have rapid antigen testing (RADT). Those at intermediate risk should have RADT. Patients determined to be high risk based on one of these tools can either have rapid testing done or can be empirically treated with antibiotics[1,16] (**Table 1**).

Testing

RADT has been validated for use with the clinical decision tools aforementioned. Another type of rapid testing that utilizes nucleic acid amplification techniques is available in the United States and is more sensitive and specific. However, it is also more expensive and more research needs to be done in conjunction with appropriate clinical decision tools in order to validate its use.

Throat culture is not indicated in the majority of adult patients but can be considered in patients who are high risk of complications such as immunocompromised patients. Both the Centers for Disease Control and Prevention (CDC) and the American Academy of Pediatrics state that children and adolescents should undergo throat culture done if RADT is negative and then be appropriately treated with antibiotics if throat culture returns positive for streptococcus due to this age group having high risk of complications including peritonsillar abscess, rheumatic fever, and poststreptococcal glomerulonephritis. However, this has not recently been found to be cost-effective in the United States due to the fact that the prevalence of rheumatic heart disease is extremely low.[1,16] If RADT is negative for GAS but the patient has severe symptoms, consider Group C or Group G streptococcus, which would require a throat culture for diagnosis of this strain.[17]

For comparison, RADT has a sensitivity of diagnosing GAS infection of 59% to 96% depending on which type is used, nucleic acid amplification testing has a sensitivity of 93% to 99%, and throat culture has a sensitivity of 90% to 95%.[1,16]

Viral testing may be of help in diagnosing pharyngitis due to COVID-19, influenza, mononucleosis, or HIV. Most primary care offices have access to point of care COVID-19 and influenza testing, which may be helpful in diagnosis and determining the etiology of viral pharyngitis. EBV and CMV testing may be performed to aid in the diagnosis of mononucleosis. EBV testing can include viral capsid antigen (VCA), early antigen, EBV nuclear antigen (EBNA), and monospot testing. Primary current EBV infection can be suspected when patients have anti-VCA immunoglobulin M (IgM) but do not have antibodies to EBNA or if patients have high or increasing levels of anti-VCA IgG and no antibodies to EBNA. Past infection is evidenced by antibodies to both VCA and EBNA. In general, monospot testing is not recommended by the CDC as there are often false negatives and false positives, and it is not a very accurate test in children as the antibodies that monospot tests for are often not present in children infected by EBV. A CBC may also be helpful in mononucleosis as it will often show lymphocytosis with atypical lymphocytes at levels of 10% or more.[18] Mononucleosis caused by CMV is best diagnosed by a positive IgM serology.[14]

Pharyngitis as a result of candida infection is usually a clinical diagnosis. If it persists despite treatment, cultures and sensitivities may be helpful. If the lesion can be visualized, a microbial culture can be taken of the lesion. If there is no visible lesion but

Table 1
Clinical decision tools substantiated specifically for streptococcal pharyngitis

Criteria	Centor	McIsaac/ Modified Centor	Fever-PAIN
Lack of cough	+1	+1	+1
Tonsillar exudate or swelling	+1	+1	Not applicable
Fever (≥100.4°F)	+1	+1	+1
Swollen, tender anterior cervical chain lymphadenopathy	+1	+1	Not applicable
Age	Not applicable	3–14 y = +1 15–44 y = 0 ≥45 y = −1	Not applicable
Purulent tonsils	Not applicable	Not applicable	+1
Intensely inflamed tonsils	Not applicable	Not applicable	+1
Presentation within 3 d of symptom onset	Not applicable	Not applicable	+1
Risk score	1–1, low risk; 2–3, intermediate risk; 4–5, high risk		

candida is considered to be a likely diagnosis, a whole saliva sample can be taken. If dentures are involved, a sample should also be taken from both the dentures and the palate.[15]

Laryngoscopy and pH monitoring are the tests currently available to test for LPR. However, they are notably inaccurate and often miss the diagnosis. A trial of PPIs is considered both diagnostic and therapeutic in many cases.[11]

TREATMENT
Infectious Causes

Viral pathogens
The mainstay of treatment in viral pharyngitis cases is supportive therapy. In certain specific viral illnesses such as influenza A and B, severe acute respiratory syndrome coronavirus 2 (SARS-CoV-2), and herpes simplex viruses, specific antiviral therapies can be used, which may help reduce the severity and length of illness. For influenza A and B, oseltamivir, zanamivir, peramivir, or baloxavir can be prescribed. Tamiflu is the only anti-influenza agent approved for use in infants and children aged 14 days to 7 years, while zanamivir is indicated in adults and children aged 7 years and older, peramivir is indicated in adults and children aged 13 years and older, and baloxavir is indicated in adults and children aged 12 years and older.[19] Pharyngitis can be a presenting symptom in oral mucocutaneous herpes simplex infections, and appropriate antiviral therapy with acyclovir, valacyclovir, famciclovir, or ganciclovir will improve the associated sore throat.[20] Antiviral therapy has not been shown to be effective in EBV-induced and CMV-induced infectious mononucleosis, and first-line recommended treatment is supportive therapy only with close monitoring for complications.[14] Acute onset upper respiratory symptoms including fever, nonexudative pharyngitis, and diffuse adenopathy in patients with history of high-risk sexual behavior is concerning for acute HIV infection and requires appropriate testing and treatment if this diagnosis is confirmed.[17]

Supportive

Supportive therapies to consider include NSAIDs, acetaminophen, corticosteroids, topical anesthetics, medicated throat lozenges, and salt water gargles.[1,16] NSAIDs have proven to be more effective in reducing tonsillar swelling while also managing pain and fever compared to acetaminophen.[16] While corticosteroids are effective in reducing pain and swelling, these medications carry increased risk of side effects compared to NSAIDs, which resulted in guidelines advising against corticosteroid use in pharyngitis. However, more recent studies demonstrate that a single dose of a high-potency corticosteroid such as dexamethasone, administered within 24 hours of onset of symptoms, is more effective in rapidly reducing pain and swelling compared to NSAIDs alone in patients aged 5 years and older with GAS pharyngitis. The suggested dose for dexamethasone in GAS cases is 0.6 mg/kg (maximum dose 10 mg) by mouth.[1] Intravenous or intramuscular corticosteroid therapy is recommended in all cases of airway compromise in the setting of pharyngitis. Topical anesthetics and medicated throat lozenges are effective in reducing pain but require frequent redosing approximately every 2 hours.

Bacterial pathogens

Oral penicillin V potassium remains the first-line therapeutic agent recommended for the treatment of GAS pharyngitis. Given the low cost, minimal side effect profile, and the ongoing sensitivity of GAS to this agent, penicillin is considered a safe and effective treatment option.[1,16] Amoxicillin is an equally effective alternative with the benefit of available liquid formulations for patients who cannot tolerate tablets. A single intramuscular dose of penicillin G benzathine is another alternative therapy. For patients with type IV hypersensitivity reactions (ie, rash) to penicillin, cephalosporins (eg, cephalexin) are effective and safe. In the case of more severe penicillin allergic reactions such as anaphylaxis (type 1 hypersensitivity), macrolides such as azithromycin and clarithromycin, or oral clindamycin are recommended therapies. With the exception of azithromycin, which requires a 5 day course of therapy, all oral antibiotics noted here require a 10 day course of treatment. Antibiotic treatment of group C and G streptococcal pharyngitis is not recommended as these non-GAS infections do not progress to rheumatic fever; however, antibiotic therapy may reduce pain.[1] Appropriate antibiotic therapy should be initiated in the setting of positive RADT and/or throat culture results. Patients with streptococcal bacterial pharyngitis should not be cleared to return to school or work until fever has resolved and/or a minimum of 24 hours of antibiotic therapy has been completed. Patients with GAS pharyngitis require re-evaluation if symptoms worsen despite 5 days of appropriate treatment. Hospitalization is indicated in cases of sepsis, airway compromise, need for intravenous antibiotic therapy, and/or suspicion for Lemierre syndrome.

Gonococcal pharyngitis treatment regimens are the same as gonococcal genitourinary infections. Patients should receive intramuscular ceftriaxone along with oral doxycycline or azithromycin to reduce the risk of resistance and because there is 20% to 54% rate of coinfection with chlamydia.[8] Sexual contact should be avoided until therapy is completed and symptoms have resolved, and patients should be counseled regarding the need for condom use with all sexual contact.

Fungal pathogens

Fungal pharyngitis, most commonly caused by C albicans, should be treated with either oral nystatin solution for 7 to 10 days or fluconazole 100 to 200 mg tablet daily for 7 to 14 days.[21] If inhaled corticosteroid use is the suspected precipitating factor, education regarding rinsing mouth after inhaler use should be provided.

Surgical management

Definitive surgical intervention with tonsillectomy should be considered in patients with a high frequency of recurrent GAS or other bacterial pharyngitis, those with multiple antibiotic allergies complicating management, or those with a history of serious complications such as peritonsillar abscess.[1,16] When considering surgical intervention, clinicians should be cognizant that the risk and incidence of bacterial pharyngitis decreases with age, especially in patients aged older than 10 years.[16] High frequency of recurrence is generally defined as 7 episodes in a 1 year period, 5 episodes per year over a 2 year period, or 3 episodes per year over a 3 year period.[1] While tonsillectomy does reduce the risk of tonsillitis, studies have only demonstrated moderate long-term benefit in reducing recurrent sore throat/pharyngitis episodes.[22]

Noninfectious Causes

Trauma

Definitive treatment of trauma-induced pharyngitis includes removal or resolution of the inciting trauma while providing supportive care until symptoms resolve. In the case of postoperative pharyngitis, the risk of occurrence can be reduced with the use of inhaled fluticasone propionate, intravenous dexamethasone, and lidocaine. Additionally, the use of topical NSAIDs, lozenges, and ketamine gargles postoperatively reduce pain and swelling.[3] Addressing the underlying cause of the turbulent airflow in snoring-induced pharyngitis is the preferred treatment, but supportive therapies provide symptomatic relief while diagnostic workup and treatment plans are developed. Sore throats due to excessive talking or yelling should be managed with voice rest and supportive therapies.

Irritants

Avoidance of irritants or allergens causing pharyngitis is the primary treatment in these cases. For instance, smoking cessation counseling should be provided to those using cigarettes, pipes, cigars, hookah, electronic cigarettes, and inhaled marijuana.[3,9,10]

For allergen-induced pharyngitis, reducing the risk of exposure to inciting allergens is recommended when possible. However, for common seasonal and environmental allergens such as pollen, grass, ragweed, and dust mites, this is not realistic. While maintaining a clean home environment is recommended to reduce dust mite exposure, evidence has not demonstrated a reduction in allergy symptoms and the need for medication with the use of dust mite-proof mattresses, pillows, quilt covers or similar products, and high-efficiency particulate air filters. Age-appropriate treatment of allergic rhinitis with associated pharyngitis is recommended. Treatment options include intranasal corticosteroids, oral antihistamines, intranasal antihistamines, combined intranasal corticosteroid and antihistamine formulations, oral decongestants, intranasal cromolyn, intranasal ipratropium, and leukotriene receptor antagonists. Of note, when selecting allergy treatments, clinicians must consider that intranasal corticosteroids, antihistamines, and combined corticosteroid-antihistamine formulations can potentially cause pharyngitis.[23]

Laryngopharyngeal reflux

LPR-induced pharyngitis treatment is focused on addressing the underlying gastroesophageal reflux and should include the elimination of inciting foods, weight loss, smoking cessation, limiting/eliminating alcohol, and avoiding food intake prior to bedtime. Additional treatment options include pharmacologic therapy with PPIs or combined PPIs and histamine 2-receptor antagonists for cases resistant to PPIs alone. Surgical intervention with Nissen fundoplication may be indicated in patients who do not respond to pharmacologic therapy; however, outcome studies have resulted in conflicting evidence as to whether this treatment is effective in resolving LPR resistant to PPI therapy. The proposed reasoning for these variable outcomes is misdiagnosis of LPR as the cause of pharyngitis resulting in a lack of response to PPI therapy and no improvement following surgery.[11]

Medications
Medication-induced pharyngitis treatment includes discontinuation or substitution of inciting medications if clinically appropriate, and/or supportive therapies. In cases of pill esophagitis with associated pharyngitis, patients should be educated regarding the need to take potentially problematic medications with a full glass of water while sitting upright and remaining upright for 30 minutes after medication administration.[12]

EMERGING THERAPIES

During and following the 2020 COVID-19 pandemic, pharyngitis cases due to infection with SARS-CoV-2 dramatically increased. This viral pharyngitis can be appropriately treated with antiviral therapies approved in the treatment of COVID-19 and include oral nirmatrelvir/ritonavir and intravenous remdesivir.[24] Patients who do not meet criteria for these pharmacologic therapies should be treated with supportive therapies previously discussed.

Another emerging clinical trend now widely accepted following the COVID-19 pandemic is the use of telemedicine in evaluating and treating patients with pharyngitis. While patients can provide equivalent history in both face-to-face and telemedicine visits, caution should be exercised when prescribing antibiotics for GAS pharyngitis following telemedicine encounters due to the limitations of effective patient self-examination. Studies show that patients overreport tonsillar exudate, erythema, and tender anterior cervical lymphadenitis, and patients have difficulty providing clinically useful oropharyngeal images. This imprecision in self-examination may result in falsely elevated clinical decision tool scores that can lead to inappropriate empiric antibiotic therapy.[1] The risks versus benefits of antibiotic use should be carefully considered and discussed with patients when assessing pharyngitis via telemedicine encounters.

COMPLICATIONS

The majority of serious pharyngitis complications is observed in GAS pharyngitis and includes the development of antibiotic resistance, adverse reactions to antibiotics, epiglottitis, peritonsillar abscess, retropharyngeal abscess, rheumatic fever and heart disease, poststreptococcal glomerulonephritis, and Lemierre syndrome.[1,16] Lemierre syndrome is an extension of bacterial pharyngitis into the lateral pharyngeal space with the development of jugular vein thrombophlebitis resulting in bacteremia and sepsis. Lemierre syndrome is a known complication of GAS infection, but the primary cause is *F necrophorum* pharyngitis.[6] Serious complications resulting from GAS pharyngitis are more common in children and adolescents; therefore, the threshold to initiate antibiotic therapy in this population should be lower as conditions such as peritonsillar abscess, rheumatic fever, and poststreptococcal glomerulonephritis can be avoided with initiation of appropriate antibiotic therapy within 9 days of onset of symptoms.[16] In the United States, rheumatic fever has an estimated incidence of 0.5 episodes per 100,000 people with rheumatic heart disease occurring in 50% to 70% of rheumatic fever cases.[1]

In all cases of pharyngitis, complications include loss of productivity (absence from work), education setbacks (absence from school), social isolation, and adverse reactions to therapies. Prompt and accurate diagnosis of pharyngitis etiology followed by appropriate management reduces the risk of these complications. Of particular concern is the overuse of antibiotics in pharyngitis cases. Antibiotic use, both appropriate and inappropriate, increases the risk of resistance development, adverse reactions including allergic reactions, *Clostridium difficile* colitis (especially with clindamycin use), and increased financial burden on patients and the health care system.

RECURRENCE MANAGEMENT

When bacterial pharyngitis cases do not respond to appropriate antibiotic therapy or there is recurrence, high suspicion for misdiagnosis should exist and consideration be given to possible viral or noninfectious etiologies. If antibiotic therapy was initiated on the basis of RADT results alone, a throat culture should be obtained to confirm diagnosis as well as antibiotic sensitivity.

Confirmed recurrence or persistence of bacterial pharyngitis, particularly GAS pharyngitis, is most often due to noncompliance with or nonadherence to the treatment course, but antibiotic resistance should be considered. For GAS pharyngitis, in patients initially treated with a 10 day course of penicillin, recurrent cases can be effectively managed with amoxicillin/clavulanate, clindamycin, or intramuscular penicillin G benzathine. Patients with penicillin allergies who were initially managed with a first-generation cephalosporin can be treated with a third-generation cephalosporin.[1,16] When recurrence of viral pharyngitis occurs, consideration should be given to superimposed bacterial etiology or some other noninfectious cause. Infectious pharyngitis, particularly bacterial cases, are contagious; therefore, toothbrushes should be changed and dentures, retainers, and other oral devices thoroughly cleansed and disinfected within 24 to 48 hours after initiation of treatment to prevent reinfection.

Emerging evidence reveals that approximately 10% of bacterial pharyngitis cases in adolescents and young adults are due to *F necrophorum*, an obligate anaerobic gram-negative bacillus.[6] Patients presenting with worsening symptoms, such as rigors, night sweats, and unilateral pain despite appropriate antibiotic therapy for GAS, should be evaluated for Lemierre syndrome.[1] This diagnosis requires prompt hospitalization for imaging, intravenous antibiotic therapy, and polymerase chain reaction testing for *F necrophorum* as this organism is the most common cause of Lemierre syndrome.[1,6]

SUMMARY

While pharyngitis is a common primary care complaint, evidence reveals that this diagnosis is an area where antibiotic therapy is frequently misused. Appropriate diagnosis and management of pharyngitis is crucial to ensure antimicrobial stewardship and improve patient safety and outcomes. Pharyngitis etiologies include both infectious and noninfectious sources such as bacteria, viruses, fungal organisms, trauma, irritants, LPR, and medications. Clinicians need to obtain a thorough history and careful physical examination, along with appropriate diagnostic testing when indicated, to ensure treatment plans are targeted toward the most likely pharyngitis etiology.

CLINICS CARE POINTS

- History combined with physical and risk score calculators should be used to increase the accuracy of testing and diagnosis of pharyngitis.

- The majority of pharyngitis is nonbacterial in etiology, and providers should practice cautious antibiotic stewardship when managing these cases.
- Practitioners should emphasize conservative management in adults and more proactive empiric treatment in pediatric patients.

DISCLOSURE

The authors have nothing to disclose.

REFERENCES

1. Hamilton JL, McCrea IIL. Streptococcal pharyngitis: rapid evidence review. Am Fam Physician 2024;109(4):343–9. Available at: https://www.aafp.org/pubs/afp/issues/2024/0400/streptococcal-pharyngitis.html.
2. Sykes EA, Wu V, Beyea MM, et al. Pharyngitis. Can Fam Physician 2020;66: 251–7. PMID: 32273409; PMCID: PMC7145142.
3. Renner B, Mueller CA, Shephard A. Environmental and non-infectious factors in the aetiology of pharyngitis (sore throat). Inflamm Res 2012;61:1041–52.
4. Wolford RW, Goyal A, Syed SYB, et al. Pharyngitis. StatPearls [Internet]. StatPearls Publishing; 2023. Available at: https://www.ncbi.nlm.nih.gov/books/NBK519550/. Accessed April 29, 2024.
5. Shulman ST, Bisno AL, Clegg HW, et al. Clinical practice guideline for the diagnosis and management of group a streptococcal pharyngitis: 2012 update by the infectious diseases society of America. Clin Infect Dis 2012; 55(10):e86–102.
6. Centor RM, Atkinson TP, Ratliff AE, et al. The clinical presentation of fusobacterium-positive and streptococcal-positive pharyngitis in a University Health Clinic. Ann Intern Med 2015;162:241–7.
7. World Health Organization. WHO delivers medicines as diphtheria spreads in Yemen. 2017. Available at: http://www.who.int/mediacentre/news/releases/2017/medicines-diphtheria-yemen/en/. Accessed April 24, 2024.
8. Herring K, Shmerling A. Case report: gonorrhea as a cause of exudative tonsillitis. Am Fam Physician 2019;99(2):77. Available at: https://www.aafp.org/pubs/afp/issues/2019/0115/p77.html.
9. Esteban-Lopez M, Perry MD, Garbinski LD, et al. Health effects and known pathology associated with the use of E-cigarettes. Toxicol Rep 2022;9:1357–68.
10. Tetrault JM, Crothers K, Moore BA, et al. Effects of marijuana smoking on pulmonary function and respiratory complications: a systematic review. Arch Intern Med 2007;167(3):221–8.
11. Campagnolo AM, Priston J, Theon RH, et al. Laryngopharyngeal reflux: diagnosis, treatment, and latest research. Int Arch Otorhinolaryngol 2014;18:184–91.
12. Kikendall JW. Pill-inducted esophagitis. Gastroenterol Hepatol 2007;3(4):275–6. PMCID: PMC3099275. PMID: 21960840.
13. Ishii T, Sasaki Y, Maeda T, et al. Clinical differentiation of infectious mononucleosis that is caused by Epstein-Barr virus or cytomegalovirus: a single-center case-control study in Japan. J Infect Chemother 2019;25(6):431–6.
14. Sylvester J, Buchanan BK, Silva TW. Infectious mononucleosis: rapid evidence review. Am Fam Physician 2023;107(1):71–8. Available at: https://www.aafp.org/pubs/afp/issues/2023/0100/infectious-mononucleosis.html.

15. Taylor M, Brizuela M, Raja A. Oral Candidiasis. *StatPearls [Internet]*. StatPearls Publishing; 2023. Available at: https://www.ncbi.nlm.nih.gov/books/NBK545282/. Accessed April 30, 2024.
16. Kalra MG, Higgins KE, Perez ED. Common questions about streptococcal pharyngitis. Am Fam Physician 2016;94(1):24–31. Available at: https://www.aafp.org/pubs/afp/issues/2016/0701/p24.html.
17. Weber R. Pharyngitis. Prim Care Clin Off Pract 2014;41(1):91–8.
18. CDC. Laboratory testing for Epstein-Barr virus (EBV). Centers for Disease Control and Prevention; 2024. Available at: https://www.cdc.gov/epstein-barr/php/laboratories/index.html. Accessed April 30, 2024.
19. Gaitonde DY, Moore FC, Morgan MK. Influenza: diagnosis and treatment. Am Fam Physician 2019;100(12):751–8. Available at: https://www.aafp.org/pubs/afp/issues/2019/1215/p751.html.
20. McMillan JA, Weiner LB, Higgins AM, et al. Pharyngitis associated with herpes simplex virus in college students. Pediatr Infect Dis J 1993;12(4):280–4.
21. Pappas PG, Krauffman CA, Andes DR, et al. Clinical practice guideline for the management of Candidiasis: 2016 Update by IDSA. Clin Infect Dis 2016;62(4):e1–50.
22. Burton MJ, Galsziou PP, Chong LY, et al. Tonsillectomy or adenotonsillectomy versus non-surgical treatment for chronic/recurrent acute tonsillitis. Cochrane Database Syst Rev 2014;(11):CD001802.
23. Weaver-Agostini J, Kosak Z, Bartlett S. Allergic rhinitis: rapid evidence review. Am Fam Physician 2023;107(5):466–73. Available at: https://www.aafp.org/pubs/afp/issues/2023/0500/allergic-rhinitis.html.
24. Cheng AM, Dollar E, Angier H. Outpatient management of COVID-19: rapid evidence review. Am Fam Physician 2023;107(4):370–81. Available at: https://www.aafp.org/pubs/afp/issues/2023/0400/outpatient-management-of-covid-19.html#afp20230400p370-f1.

Bell's Palsy

Sarah N. Dalrymple, MD, Jessica H. Row, MD,
John D. Gazewood, MD, MSPH*

KEYWORDS

- Bell's palsy • Bell palsy • Idiopathic facial nerve palsy • Peripheral facial palsy

KEY POINTS

- Bell's palsy is a common, idiopathic condition causing acute onset of unilateral facial paralysis in the distribution of peripheral cranial nerve VII.
- Diagnose Bell's palsy based on a careful history and physical examination.
- Treat all adult patients with Bell's palsy with oral corticosteroids to increase rates of complete recovery.
- Treat all adult patients with Bell's palsy with antiviral agents to reduce rates of synkinesis.
- Refer patients with incomplete recovery to physical therapy and to an appropriate specialist.

INTRODUCTION

Bell's palsy, also referred to as idiopathic facial paralysis, is an acute weakness or paralysis of the facial muscles related to swelling of the facial nerve and has no apparent cause. Primary care physicians play a pivotal in the clinical evaluation, diagnosis, treatment, and follow-up of patients with Bell's palsy, and can manage most patients with Bell's palsy in the primary care setting. This review will provide an evidence-based approach to the diagnosis and management of Bell's palsy.

EPIDEMIOLOGY

The estimated annual incidence of Bell's palsy is 20 to 30 per 100,000 people. Although the highest incidence occurs in individuals between 15 and 45 years of age, it can occur at any age.[1–4] Women and men are equally affected,[1,2] and both sides of the face are equally affected.[3,5] Conditions associated with increased risk of Bell's Palsy include diabetes,[2,6] pregnancy,[1,7] hypertension,[2] immunosuppression,[2] influenza A, and other upper respiratory illnesses.[3,5]

Department of Family Medicine, University of Virginia Health, Charlottesville, VA, USA
* Corresponding author. Department of Family Medicine, POB 8000729, UVA Health, Charlottesville, VA 22908.
E-mail address: Jdg3k@uvahealth.org

Prim Care Clin Office Pract 52 (2025) 111–121
https://doi.org/10.1016/j.pop.2024.09.012
primarycare.theclinics.com
0095-4543/25/© 2024 Elsevier Inc. All rights reserved, including those for text and data mining, AI training, and similar technologies.

PATHOGENESIS

While Bell's palsy has no apparent cause, the pathophysiology is associated with nerve edema and subsequent mechanical compression of the facial nerve, leading to weakness or paralysis in the distribution of the facial nerve (**Fig. 1**). Bell's palsy may also affect the sensory and autonomic function of the facial nerve. The facial nerve carries sensation from the external auditory canal, pinna, mastoid, and the palatal mucosa. Impaired function of the chorda tympani branch can affect taste and cause abnormal salivation. Damage to the petrosal nerve branch, which innervates the lacrimal glands, leads to decreased lacrimation. As fibers from the facial nerve also innervate the stapedius, some patients may have hyperacusis.[8,9] Potential etiologies include ischemic neuritis or reactivation of Herpes Simplex Virus Type 1 in the geniculate ganglion.[8]

CORONAVIRUS DISEASE 2019 AND BELL'S PALSY

With the onset of the coronavirus disease 2019 (COVID-19) pandemic, questions arose regarding the relationship between Bell's palsy, COVID-19 infection, and vaccinations against COVID-19. A systematic review and meta-analyses analyzed

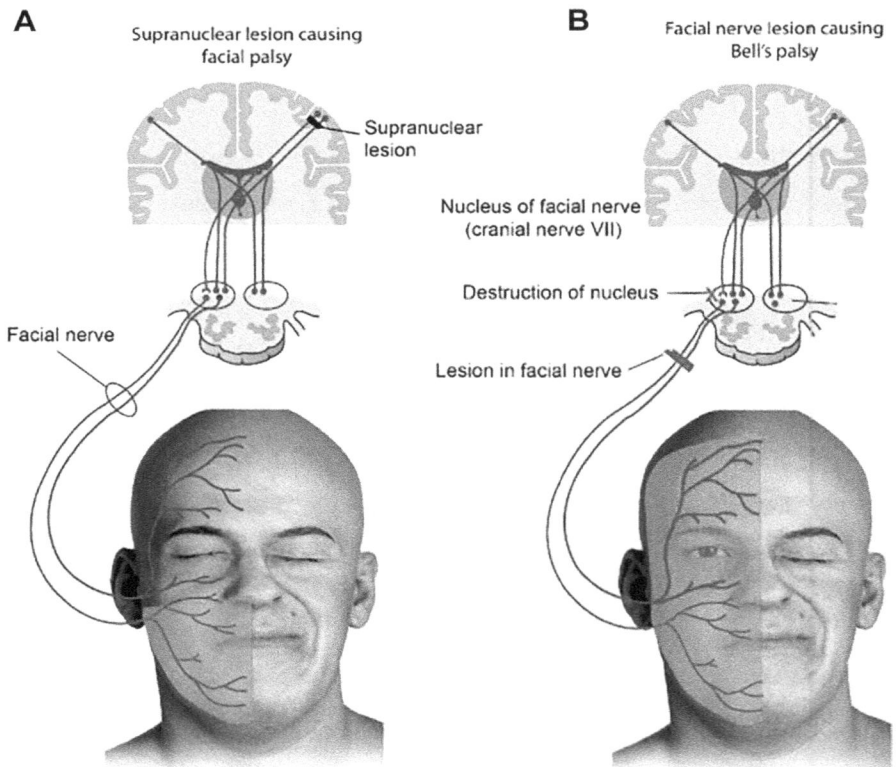

Fig. 1. Etiology of facial palsy. (*A*) Supranuclear lesion causing upper motor nerve palsy. (*B*) Facial nerve lesion causing lower motor nerve palsy, consistent with Bell's palsy. (S. M. Balaji, Padma Preetha Balaji, Chapter 40 - Sensory and motor disturbances of the orofacial region, Textbook of Oral and Maxillofacial Surgery, 4th Edition. Elsevier India, 2022.)

randomized controlled trial data and observational data. There was an increased incidence of Bell's palsy among individuals receiving either a messenger-RNA (m-RNA) vaccine or a viral vector vaccine in randomized placebo controlled-trials of both vaccine types (odds ratio [OR] 3.0, 95% confidence of interval [CI], 1.1–8.18).[10] A pooled analysis of observational studies of m-RNA vaccines, which included 13,518,026 observed doses and 13,510,701 unvaccinated individuals showed no association between vaccine administration and Bell's palsy (OR 0.7, 95% CI, 0.42–1.16).[9] This data suggest an association between COVID vaccination and incident Bell's palsy, but does not prove a causal relationship. Furthermore, Bell's palsy was observed to be more common following infection with COVID-19 than following vaccination (OR 3.23; 95% CI, 1.57–6.62).[10]

CLINICAL PRESENTATION

Bell's palsy presents acutely with unilateral facial weakness or paralysis involving the forehead developing over 24 to 48 h.[4,8] Rarely, Bell's palsy can be bilateral. The palsy most noticeably affects the motor function of the facial nerve but affects the autonomic and sensory function as well.[8] Patients may complain of alteration in taste, sensation, or hearing on the affected side.[8] The history and physical examination are essential to the diagnosis of Bell's palsy and can reliably lead to the diagnosis, as well as identify findings that raise concern for an alternative and potentially more serious diagnosis. The examiner should find no other neurologic abnormalities in addition to findings consistent with peripheral facial nerve involvement.[4,8]

EXAMINATION

Bell's palsy presents with drooping of the mouth, flattening of the nasolabial fold, inability to close the affected eye, and smoothing of the brow on the affected side.[8,9] (see **Figs. 1** and **2**) The provider should perform complete neurologic and otolaryngologic examinations with the primary goal of differentiating between an upper, or central, and lower, or peripheral, motor neuron lesion affecting the facial nerve.[11–13] By

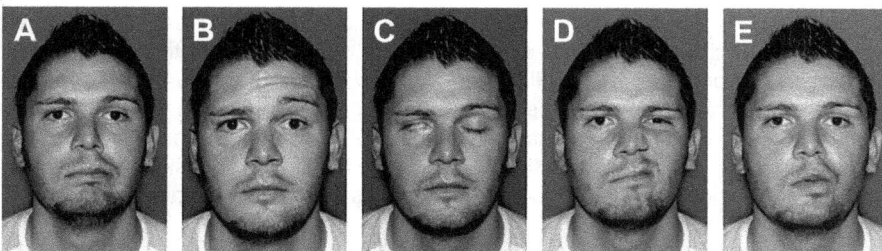

Fig. 2. Peripheral facial nerve palsy on the right side. Typical presentation of peripheral paralysis of the facial nerve (cranial nerve VII) on the right side. (*A*) Face at rest. The skin creases in the right half of the face have smoothed out. (*B*) When the patient attempts to raise his eyebrows, only the left half of the forehead displays wrinkles, due to loss of function of right frontalis muscle. (*C*) When the patient attempts to shut both eyes, he is unable to do so on the right side (lagopthhalmos) due to loss of function of the right orbicularis oculi muscle. (*D*) When patient attempts to wrinkle his nose, he is unable to do so on the right side of face. (*E*) When patient tries to whistle, no tone is produced but air escapes through the lips on the paralyzed side, due to loss of function of the orbicularis oris muscle. (Paulsen, Waschke, Sobotta Atlas of Human Anatomy, 17th Edition. 2023 © Elsevier GmbH, Urban & Fischer, Munich.)

definition, Bell's palsy is a peripheral lesion, which causes weakness of all the muscles involved in facial expression on the affected side. This includes the frontalis muscle which raises the eyebrow; orbicularis oculi muscle which closes the eyelids and is involved in tear production and the corneal reflex; the orbicularis oris muscle which closes and protracts the lips, is involved with speech, and is essential to swallowing, chewing, and sucking; the buccinator muscle which pulls the corners of the mouth laterally; and the platysma muscle which pulls down the mandible and pulls the corners of the lips out to the side and down.[8,9]

If the patient can raise their eyebrow on the affected side, suggesting that the frontalis muscle is not affected, consider a central lesion, particularly a stroke. Additionally, consider an alternative diagnosis if the initial examination reveals any neurologic findings in addition to those associated with the facial muscles described earlier as these findings would indicate a lesion affecting structures other than just cranial nerve VII.[8,9] (see **Fig. 1**) If the patient presents with ipsilateral recurrent Bell's palsy,[14] symptoms continue to progress beyond the initial 72 h after onset, the symptoms fluctuate, or there is bilateral involvement at initial presentation, additional evaluation is required.[15]

While Bell's palsy is defined as idiopathic facial nerve palsy, there are many conditions that cause peripheral facial nerve palsy or central processes that cause facial weakness. Findings that suggest an alternative diagnosis include gradual symptom onset, recent tick or vaccine exposure, tinnitus, hearing loss or vertigo, signs of infection, head and neck cancer, and limb or bulbar weakness.[8,9] Central causes will typically spare the forehead. Gradual onset and mental status changes suggest brain tumor, either primary, or if a history of cancer, metastatic. Abrupt onset associated with ipsilateral extremity weakness or other neurologic symptoms indicate a stroke. Multiple sclerosis causing facial weakness is also associated with other neurologic symptoms. Viral diseases that cause peripheral nerve palsy include COVID-19, cytomegalovirus, Epstein-Barr virus, herpes simplex, human immunodeficiency virus (HIV), influenza, mumps, and rubella—weakness associated with these infections will typically be preceded or accompanied by the associated viral syndrome. Ramsay Hunt syndrome, due to herpes zoster, is characterized by prodromal pain and a vesicular eruption in the ear canal and/or palate. Otitis media can cause peripheral nerve palsy of gradual onset, associated with pain, fever, and conductive hearing loss. Suspect Lyme disease if there is a history of tick exposure, residence in or travel to endemic areas, rash and/or arthralgias or bilateral facial weakness. Autoimmune or granulomatous conditions such as sarcoidosis, myasthenia gravis, or Guillain-Barre syndrome are more often bilateral at presentation. Cholesteatoma and head and neck cancers will typically have a gradual onset and associated findings on physical examination. Weakness associated with tinnitus and hearing loss suggests the diagnosis of acoustic neuroma.[4,8,9]

DIAGNOSTIC TESTING

Laboratory testing is not required to diagnose Bell's palsy. The provider should consider laboratory testing if the patient's history suggests an identifiable cause of peripheral facial nerve palsy, such as Lyme disease, HIV, or sarcoidosis. One guideline suggests obtaining a complete blood count with differential as an increased neutrophil-to-lymphocyte ratio has been associated with poor prognosis. However, the review upon which this recommendation is based demonstrated evidence of publication bias and was unable to provide a clear cut-off separating patients with poor prognosis from those with good prognosis.[13,16]

Imaging is not required to diagnose Bell's palsy if the physical examination findings are consistent with the diagnosis. There is a small risk of lacunar infarct affecting the lower pons that presents as a peripheral palsy; this is exceedingly rare.[17] Imaging is indicated if the patient presents with recurrent ipsilateral Bell's palsy, symptom progression beyond the initial 72 h following onset, fluctuate, or are bilateral. MRI head or MRI orbits/face/neck with and without intravenous contrast are the 2 recommended studies to evaluate for suspected tumor.[18]

CLINICAL ASSESSMENT TOOLS

Patients can experience a spectrum of symptom severity. Two grading scales are commonly used to classify severity, the House-Brackmann (**Fig. 3**) and Sunnybrook (**Fig. 4**) scales. Classifying severity can help provide appropriate anticipatory guidance, and aid in treatment recommendations, particularly early physical therapy for individuals with scores indicating higher severity.

PROGNOSIS

Most patients with Bell's palsy will recover completely but long-term sequelae can occur. Complete spontaneous recovery occurs in up to 85% of patients experiencing Bell's palsy within 3 weeks, with at least partial recovery in the following 3 to 6 months.[19] Regarding special populations, up to 90% of pregnant patients and children under the age of 14 will experience complete spontaneous recovery.[7,20] Clinically useful indicators of poor prognosis for complete spontaneous recovery include bilateral involvement and more severe symptoms (as determined by the Sunnybrook or House-Brackman assessments).[7,16,21] The recurrence rate of Bell's palsy has been estimated at 6.5% with a mean interval of 10 years. Of patients who experience a recurrence of Bell's palsy, approximately two-thirds subsequently achieve complete spontaneous recovery.[14]

Long-term sequelae of Bell's palsy, especially the impairment of smiling, may trigger anxiety, depression, and other severe psychologic problems.[22] Synkinesis, which is

HOUSE-BRACKMANN FACIAL NERVE GRADING SYSTEM

Grade I: Normal function
- Normal facial function in all areas

Grade II: Mild dysfunction
- Slight weakness noticeable on close inspection; may have very slight synkinesis

Grade III: Moderate dysfunction
- Obvious weakness or disfiguring asymmetry; normal symmetry and tone at rest; incomplete eye closure

Grade IV: Moderately severe dysfunction
- Obvious weakness or disfiguring asymmetry; normal symmetry and tone at rest; incomplete eye closure

Grade V: Severe dysfunction
- Only barely perceptible motion; asymmetry at rest

Grade VI: Total paralysis
- No movement

Fig. 3. House-Brackmann facial nerve grading scale. (Edward T. Bope, Rick D. Kellerman, Conn's Current Therapy 2012, 1 edition. Saunders, 2012.)

Sunnybrook Facial Grading System

Resting symmetry	Symmetry of voluntary movement	Synkinesis
Compared to normal side	Degree of muscle EXCURSION compared to normal side	Rate the degree of INVOLUNTARY MUSCLE CONTRACTION associated with each expression

Resting symmetry — Compared to normal side

Eye (choose one only)
- normal 0
- narrow 1
- wide 1
- eyelid surgery 1

Cheek (nasolabial fold)
- normal 0
- absent 2
- less pronounced 1
- more pronounced 1

Mouth
- normal 0
- corner dropped 1
- corner pulled up/out 1

Resting symmetry score   Total X 5 ☐

Symmetry of voluntary movement — Degree of muscle EXCURSION compared to normal side

Scale: 1 Unable to initiate movement / 2 Initiates slight movement / 3 Initiated movement with mild excursion / 4 Movement almost complete / 5 Movement complete

Standard expressions	1	2	3	4	5	☐
Forehead wrinkle (FRO)	1	2	3	4	5	☐
Gentle eye closure (OCS)	1	2	3	4	5	☐
Open mouth smile (ZYG/RIS)	1	2	3	4	5	☐
Snarl (LLA/LLS)	1	2	3	4	5	☐
Lip pucker (OOS/OOI)	1	2	3	4	5	☐

Scale: Gross asymmetry / Severe asymmetry / Moderate asymmetry / Mild asymmetry / Normal symmetry   Total ☐

Synkinesis — Rate the degree of INVOLUNTARY MUSCLE CONTRACTION associated with each expression

Scale: NONE: No synkinesis or mass movement 0 / MILD: Slight synkinesis 1 / MODERATE: Obvious but not disfiguring synkinesis 2 / SEVERE: Disfiguring synkinesis; gross mass movement of several muscles 3

0	1	2	3	☐
0	1	2	3	☐
0	1	2	3	☐
0	1	2	3	☐
0	1	2	3	☐

Patient's name _____

Dx _____

Date _____

Voluntary movement score: Total X 4 ☐

Synkinesis score: Total ☐

Vol mov't score ☐ − Resting symmetry score ☐ − Synk score ☐ = Composite score ☐

Fig. 4. Sunnybrook grading scale. (Helen Hartley, Wendy Blumenow, Rebecca Williams, Adel Fattah, 7 - Assessment and Grading of Synkinesis and Facial Palsy, Editor(s): Babak Azizzadeh, Charles Nduka, Management of Post-Facial Paralysis Synkinesis, Elsevier, 2022.)

caused by misdirection of regenerating nerve fibers, can have motor and autonomic manifestations in patients with Bell's palsy. Motor symptoms include involuntary blinking when smiling and involuntary lip movement with blinking. Autonomic symptoms can include gustatory eye watering (crocodile tears) and gustatory sweating. When severe, synkinesis can be associated with facial muscle spasm.[8] Synkinesis can affect up to 26% of patients 1 year after Bell' Palsy onset.[3]

CURRENT CONTROVERSIES

No guidelines currently recommend surgery, although all note that there is disagreement among experts regarding this recommendation.[11–13] There are 2 approaches to surgical decompression of the facial nerve, the transmastoid decompression (TMD) approach and the middle fossa decompression (MFD) approach. The theoretic rationale for surgery is that it reduces pressure, and thus ischemia, on the facial nerve in cases of severe or complete paralysis, which will lead to improved recovery. Three recent systematic reviews provide conflicting conclusions regarding the effectiveness of surgical approaches. A 2020 Cochrane review of 2 controlled trials (1 randomized, 1 quasi-randomized) showed no improvement in long-term outcomes of patients undergoing surgery compared to those having standard medical therapy.[23] A 2019 systematic review and meta-analysis, which included 5 studies excluded from the Cochrane review for methodologic flaws, showed that surgery had a positive effect.[24] Another systematic review of 7 cohort studies found that the TMD approach was no better than standard medical therapy, but that early surgery via the MFD approach (within 14 d of onset) was associated with improved outcomes.[25] When pooling all results, no improvement for surgical intervention was found.[25] Potential adverse effects of surgery include hearing loss, tinnitus, and cerebrospinal fluid leaks, depending upon the approach.[25] Only consider surgical referral for patients with complete paralysis or severe Bell's palsy who have not responded to medical therapy. Refer these patients to advanced centers with expertise in facial nerve decompression surgery.[12]

Another area of controversy in treatment of Bell's palsy is the role of acupuncture. None of the current guidelines recommend acupuncture.[11-13] A Cochrane review found no evidence that acupuncture was beneficial.[26] A systematic review and meta-analysis found that acupuncture did show a slight benefit when added to standard therapy, but the quality of the included trials was poor and the authors did not find that the available evidence supported the use of acupuncture.[27] Well done randomized controlled trials are needed before acupuncture can be routinely offered as a safe and effective treatment modality.

MEDICAL/PHARMACOLOGIC MANAGEMENT

All patients 16 year of age and older with Bell's palsy should be treated with corticosteroids, within 72 h of onset.[11-13] Multiple randomized control trials and meta-analyses have confirmed their effectiveness in improving rates of complete recovery, with a Number Needed to Treat (NNT) = 10.[3,28,29] Less strong evidence, based on indirect comparison, suggests that a total dose of more than 450 mg for a course of steroids improves recovery rates compared to cumulative doses of 450 mg or less.[28] A typical dose studied in trials is 1 mg/kg per day of prednisone for 5 d, followed by a 5 d taper.[3,28] The French Guidelines recommend very high doses of steroids (120–200 mg/d) in severe cases.[13] A systematic review of retrospective cohort studies examining high dose versus standard dose therapy did not find improvement in outcomes (OR 0.58, 95% CI 0.27–1.22) except in those patients with severe Bell's palsy who did not receive antiviral medication (OR 0.14, 95% CI 0.04–0.54).[30] Offering patients with severe Bell's palsy who are unable to take antiviral medications a high dose of oral corticosteroids is an option for shared decision-making.

While there are limited data to guide the treatment of pregnant women with Bell's palsy, expert consensus is to treat pregnant women with oral corticosteroids.[7]

Do not offer prednisone to children. A large, randomized trial comparing oral corticosteroids to placebo among children under age 18 presenting to an emergency department showed there was no difference in recovery rates at 3 mo, 6 mo, or at 1 y, respectively, and no serious adverse events were reported.[31,32] There was no difference in response rates between children below age 12 and those 12 and older.[32] Earlier studies of oral corticosteroids and antiviral agents in adults did include adolescents aged 16 and older.[3,28,29] These disparate data should be discussed with patients and their parent or guardian to achieve a shared decision for adolescents between the ages of 16 and 18.

Offer antiviral agents to adults with Bell's palsy, in addition to corticosteroids, to reduce the risk of synkinesis. A Cochrane review provides high quality evidence that adding antiviral agents to steroids reduces the risk of synkinesis, NNT = 12.[5] Meta-analysis and network meta-analyses (NMA) provide weak evidence that combined therapy with steroids and oral antivirals reduce rates of incomplete recovery and improve patient satisfaction with recovery.[5,29] One NMA identified famciclovir as the most effective agent to combine with a steroid to improve rates of recovery.[33] This same NMA suggested that acyclovir was most effective at reducing rates of synkinesis.[33] Antivirals alone provide no benefit to patients with Bell's palsy and they should not be prescribed without corticosteroids.[11-13,34] Currently, the available evidence does not strongly support the use of one antiviral agent over another. Prescribe acyclovir, famciclovir, or valacyclovir. Dosages in studies range from 1200 mg to 2400 mg/d in divided doses for 7 to 10 d for acyclovir, 250 mg TID for 7 d for famciclovir and 500 mg BID for 5 d to 1 gm TID for 7 d for valacyclovir.

All guidelines recommend, on the strength of expert opinion, protective eye care to patients with Bell's palsy who are unable to close their eye. This consists of application of topical moisturizers, and taping the eyelid closed at bedtime, to prevent corneal damage.[11–13]

Refer patients who do not experience complete recovery to physical therapy. A 2011 Cochrane review and a more recent systematic review of randomized or quasi-randomized trials provide weak evidence that physical therapy can help patients achieve full recovery or improvement.[35,36] The available evidence does not allow for precise recommendations regarding the timing of physical therapy referral or the physical therapy regimen.

Patients with synkinesis or persistent weakness may also benefit from treatment with botulinum toxin. One review showed improvement in quality-of-life measures following treatment with Botox.[37] Another systematic review showed that Botox improves outcomes in patient with synkinesis.[38] Due to the diversity of individual patient presentations, it is not possible to recommend specific treatment regimens with Botox, in terms of type of toxin, dosage, injection site, or frequency of repetition.[38]

Available data do not support a role for hyperbaric oxygen, electrical stimulation, laser therapy, stellate ganglion blocks, or intratympanic steroid injections in the treatment of Bell's palsy.[11–13,39–41]

PATIENT MONITORING

Patients with BP should be seen periodically to assess for resolution of facial weakness and any complications, such as corneal ulceration. Refer patients to an appropriate specialist if new or worsening weakness develops, complete or severe paralysis does not improve within 1 to 2 w, eye symptoms develop, or if there is incomplete recovery at 3 mo.[11–13]

SUMMARY

Bell's palsy is characterized by abrupt onset of unilateral facial weakness and can be associated with alterations in taste or sensation, as well as hyperacusis. Laboratory testing or imaging is not needed for patients with a typical presentation. Gradual onset, sparing of the forehead, pain, and other neurologic or systemic symptoms or examination findings suggest and alternative diagnosis. The prognosis for complete recovery in Bell's palsy is good. Treat all adult patients with oral corticosteroids to increase rates of complete recovery and with oral antivirals to reduce rates of synkinesis. Refer patients with severe Bell's palsy or incomplete recovery to physical therapy, and if patients do not improve with treatment refer to an appropriate specialist.

CLINICS CARE POINTS

- Diagnose Bell's palsy based on a careful history and physical.
- Provide eye protection to all patients with Bell's palsy who cannot completely close their eye.
- Treat all adult patients with Bell's palsy with oral corticosteroids at a dose of 1 mg/kg for 5 d, followed by a 5-d taper.

- Treat all adult patients with oral acyclovir, famciclovir, or valacyclovir to reduce rates of synkinesis.
- Do not prescribe steroids or antivirals to children with Bell's palsy.

DISCLOSURE

The authors have nothing to disclose.

REFERENCES

1. Greco A, Gallo A, Fusconi M, et al. Bell's palsy and autoimmunity. Autoimmun Rev 2012;12(2):323–8. https://doi.org/10.1016/j.autrev.2012.05.008.
2. Skuladottir ATh, Bjornsdottir G, Thorleifsson G, et al. A meta-analysis uncovers the first sequence variant conferring risk of Bell's palsy. Sci Rep 2021;11:4188. https://doi.org/10.1038/s41598-021-82736-w.
3. Madhok VB, Gagyor I, Daly F, et al. Corticosteroids for Bell's palsy (idiopathic facial paralysis). Cochrane Database Syst Rev 2016;7:CD001942. https://doi.org/10.1002/14651858.CD001942.pub5.
4. Gilden DH. Clinical practice. Bell's Palsy. N Engl J Med 2004;351(13):1323–31. https://doi.org/10.1056/NEJMcp041120.
5. Gagyor I, Madhok VB, Daly F, et al. Antiviral treatment for Bell's palsy (idiopathic facial paralysis). Cochrane Database Syst Rev 2019;9:CD001869. https://doi.org/10.1002/14651858.CD001869.pub9.
6. Adour K, Wingerd J, Doty HE. Prevalence of concurrent diabetes mellitus and idiopathic facial paralysis (Bell's palsy). Diabetes 1975;24(5):449–51. https://doi.org/10.2337/diab.24.5.449.
7. Cohen Y, Lavie O, Granovsky-Grisaru S, et al. Bell palsy complicating pregnancy: a review. Obstet Gynecol Surv 2000;55(3):184–8. https://doi.org/10.1097/00006254-200003000.
8. Reich SG. Bell's palsy. Continuum 2017;23(2):447–66.
9. Dulak D, Naqvi IA. Neuroanatomy, cranial nerve 7 (Facial). In: StatPearls. Stat-Pearls Publishing; 2022. Available at: http://www.ncbi.nlm.nih.gov/books/NBK526119/. Accessed June 19, 2024.
10. Rafati A, Pasebani Y, Jameie M al. Association of SARS-CoV-2 vaccination or infection with Bell p alsy: a systematic review and meta-analysis. JAMA Otolaryngol Head Neck Surg 2023;149(6):493–504. https://doi.org/10.1001/jamaoto.2023.0160.
11. Baugh RF, Basura GJ, Ishii LE, et al. Clinical practice guideline: Bell's palsy. Otolaryngol–Head Neck Surg Off J Am Acad Otolaryngol-Head Neck Surg. 2013;149(3 Suppl):S1–27. https://doi.org/10.1177/0194599813505967.
12. de Almeida JR, Guyatt GH, Sud S, et al. Management of Bell palsy: clinical practice guideline. CMAJ Can Med Assoc J. 2014;186(12):917–22. https://doi.org/10.1503/cmaj.131801.
13. Fieux M, Franco-Vidal V, Devic P, et al. French Society of ENT (SFORL) guidelines. Management of acute Bell's palsy. Eur Ann Otorhinolaryngol Head Neck Dis 2020;137(6):483–8. https://doi.org/10.1016/j.anorl.2020.06.004.
14. Dong SH, Jung AR, Jung J, et al. Recurrent Bell's palsy. Clin Otolaryngol Off J ENT-UK Off J Neth Soc Oto-Rhino-Laryngol Cervico-Facial Surg. 2019;44(3):305–12.

15. Dalrymple SN, Row JH, Gazewood J. Bell palsy: rapid evidence review. Am Fam Physician 2023;107(4):415–20.
16. Oya R, Takenaka Y, Imai T, et al. Neutrophil-to-lymphocyte ratio and platelet-to-lymphocyte ratio as prognostic hematologic markers of Bell's palsy. A Meta-analysis Otol Neurotol 2019;40(5):681–7.
17. Bassetti C, Barth A, Regli F. Isolated infarcts of the pons. Neurology 1996;46:165–75.
18. Expert Panel on Neurologic Imaging:, Policeni B, Corey AS, et al. ACR appropriateness criteria® cranial neuropathy. J Am Coll Radiol JACR 2017;14(11S):S406–20. https://doi.org/10.1016/j.jacr.2017.08.035.
19. Peitersen E. Bell's palsy: the spontaneous course of 2,500 peripheral facial nerve palsies of different etiologies. Acta Oto-Laryngol Suppl 2002;549:4–30.
20. Pitaro J, Waissbluth S, Daniel SJ. Do children with Bell's palsy benefit from steroid treatment? A systematic review. Int J Pediatr Otorhinolaryngol 2012;76(7):921–6.
21. Calles Monar PS, Marqués Fernández VE, Sánchez-Tocino H, et al. Retrospective study of peripheral facial paralysis in a tertiary hospital over 3 years. Arch Soc Esp Oftalmol 2023;98(3):132–41.
22. Fu L, Bundy C, Sadiq SA. Psychological distress in people with disfigurement from facial palsy. Eye Lond Engl 2011;25(10):1322–6. https://doi.org/10.1038/eye.2011.158.
23. Menchetti I, McAllister K, Walker D, et al. Surgical interventions for the early management of Bell's palsy. Cochrane Database Syst Rev 2021;2021(1):CD007468. https://doi.org/10.1002/14651858.CD007468.pub4.
24. Lee SY, Seong J, Kim YH. Clinical implication of facial nerve decompression in complete Bell's palsy: a systematic review and meta-analysis. Clin Exp Otorhinolaryngol 2019;12(4):348–59.
25. Casazza GC, Schwartz SR, Gurgel RK. Systematic review of facial nerve outcomes after middle fossa decompression and transmastoid decompression for Bell's Palsy with complete facial paralysis. Otol Neurotol 2018;39(10):1311–8.
26. He L, Zhou D, Wu B, et al. Acupuncture for Bell's palsy (Cochrane review), . The Cochrane Library 2010 Issue 8. Chichester, UK: John Wiley & Sons, Ltd; 2010.
27. Li P, Qiu T, Qin C. Efficacy of acupuncture for bell's palsy: a systematic review and meta-analysis of randomized controlled trials. PLoS One 2015;10(5):e0121880.
28. de Almeida JR, Al Khabori M, Guyatt GH, et al. Combined corticosteroid and antiviral treatment for Bell palsy: a systematic review and meta-analysis. JAMA 2009;302(9):985–93. https://doi.org/10.1001/jama.2009.1243.
29. Jalali MM, Soleimani R, Soltanipour S, et al. Pharmacological treatments of bell's palsy in adults: a systematic review and network meta-analysis. Laryngoscope 2021;131(7):1615–25. https://doi.org/10.1002/lary.29368.
30. Fujiwara T, Namekawa M, Kuriyama A, et al. High-dose corticosteroids for adult Bell's palsy: systematic review and meta-analysis. Otol Neurotol 2019;40(8):1101–8.
31. Babl FE, Gerd D, Borland ML, et al. Efficacy of prednisolone for Bell palsy in children: a randomized, double-blind, placebo-controlled, multicenter trial. Neurology 2022;25. e2241ee2252.
32. Babl FE, Herd D, Borland ML, et al. Facial function in bell palsy in a Cohort of children randomized to prednisolone or placebo 12 months after diagnosis. Pediatr Neurol 2024;153:44–7. https://doi.org/10.1016/j.pediatrneurol.2024.01.011.
33. Cao J, Zhang X, Wang Z. Effectiveness comparisons of antiviral treatments for Bell palsy: a systematic review and network meta-analysis. J Neurol 2022;269(3):1353–67. https://doi.org/10.1007/s00415-021-10487-9.

34. Turgeon RD, Wilby KJ, Ensom MHH. Antiviral treatment of Bell's Palsy Based on baseline severity: a systematic review and meta-analysis. Am J Med 2015;128(6): 617–28. https://doi.org/10.1016/j.amjmed.2014.11.033.

35. Teixeira LJ, Valbuza JS, Prado GF. Physical therapy for Bell's palsy (idiopathic facial paralysis). Cochrane Database Syst Rev 2011;(12):CD006283. https://doi.org/10.1002/14651858.CD006283.pub3.

36. Ferreira M, Marques EE, Duarte JA, et al. Physical therapy with drug treatment in bell palsy: a focused review. Am J Phys Med Rehabil 2015;94:331Y340.

37. Fuzi J, Taylor A, Sideris A, et al. Does botulinum toxin therapy improve quality of life in patients with facial palsy? Aesthetic Plast Surg 2020;44:1811–9.

38. de Jongh FW, Schaeffers AW, Kooreman ZE, et al. Botulinim toxin A treatment n facial palsy synkinesis: a systematic review and meta-analalysis. Eur Arch Oto-Rhino-Laryngol 2023;280(4):1581–92.

39. Javaherian M, Attarbashi Moghaddam B, Bashardoust Tajali S, et al. Efficacy of low-level laser therapy on management of Bell's palsy: a systematic review. Laser Med Sci 2020;35(6):1245–52. https://doi.org/10.1007/s10103-020-02996-2.

40. Holland NJ, Bernstein JM, Hamilton JW. Hyperbaric oxygen therapy for Bell's palsy. Cochrane Database Syst Rev 2012;(2):CD007288. https://doi.org/10.1002/14651858.CD007288.pub2.

41. Chung JH, Park CW, Lee SH, et al. Intratympanic steroid injection for Bell's palsy: preliminary randomized controlled study. Otol Neurotol Off Publ Am Otol Soc Am Neurotol Soc Eur Acad Otol Neurotol 2014;35(9):1673–8. https://doi.org/10.1097/MAO.0000000000000505.

Vocal Cord Disorders

Bernadette Pendergraph, MD[a,b,]*, John Cheng, MD[b,c],
Claudia Alvarez, DO[d], Simran Singh, DO[e]

KEYWORDS

- Dysphonia • Vocal fold dysfunction • Hoarseness • Vocal fold nodule
- Vocal fold polyp • Voice disorder • Voice therapy

KEY POINTS

- The Clinical Practice Guideline for Hoarseness from 2018 American Academy of Otolaryngology-Head and Neck Surgery Foundation (AAO-HNSF) emphasizes no empiric treatment of dysphonia with antibiotics, anti-reflux medications, corticosteroids, or speech therapy without direct visualization of vocal folds to ensure correct diagnosis and avoid medication side effects or potential delayed diagnosis of carcinoma.
- Direct visualization of the vocal folds is necessary for dysphonia lasting more than 4 weeks.
- Voice hygiene and speech therapy are used in the treatment of most vocal fold conditions.
- Adjunct treatments for vocal fold disorders include steroid and botulinum toxin injections and potentially surgery.

INTRODUCTION

Vocal cord disorders are a diverse group of conditions that cause symptoms of hoarseness, breathing, and stridor.[1] Hoarseness is the patient's complaint of vocal dysfunction, whereas dysphonia is the clinical term for changes in voice related to altered pitch, quality, or effort.

Dysphonia is often self-limited and may be related to viral infections, but other conditions such as reflux, functional disorders, structural changes to the vocal cords, and overuse are common.[2]

The morbidity and economic costs of dysphonia are significant. From an analysis of National Health Interview Survey data, the prevalence of dysphonia among United States

[a] Harbor-UCLA Family Medicine Residency Program, Harbor-UCLA/Team to Win/Kaiser Permanente Sports Medicine Fellowship, 1403 West Lomita Boulevard Suite 105, Harbor City, CA 90710, USA; [b] Department of Family Medicine, David Geffen School of Medicine at UCLA, Los Angeles, CA 90095, USA; [c] Harbor-UCLA Family Medicine Clinic, Harbor-UCLA Medical Center, 1403 West Lomita Boulevard Suite 102, Harbor City, CA 90710, USA; [d] Family Medicine Residency Faculty, Department of Family Medicine, Harbor-UCLA Medical Center, 1403 West Lomita Boulevard Suite 102, Harbor City, CA 90710, USA; [e] Department of Family Medicine, Morehouse School of Medicine, California Hospital Medical Center Residency, 1401 South grand Avenue Leavy Hall 413, Los Angeles, CA 90015, USA
* Corresponding author.
E-mail address: bpendergraph@dhs.lacounty.gov

Prim Care Clin Office Pract 52 (2025) 123–137
https://doi.org/10.1016/j.pop.2024.09.013
primarycare.theclinics.com
0095-4543/25/© 2024 Elsevier Inc. All rights reserved, including those for text and data mining, AI training, and similar technologies.

(US) adults in the preceding 12 mo has increased from 17.89 million (7.62%) in 2012 to 29.92 million adults (11.71%) in 2022. Young adults 18 to 29 years old, women, non-Hispanic, and non-Caucasian were all more likely to report dysphonia.[3] An estimated 28 million people experience voice disorders daily in the US, with 7.2% missing at least 1 workday annually and 10% filing for short-term disability.[4] Those who file for short-term disability lost a mean of 39.2 days of work, with a mean of $4437.89 in lost wages.[5] Quality-of-life decreases are significant in those who depend on their voice, resulting in lost productivity, social isolation, and depression. While often self-limited, treatment costs about $13.5 billion annually, comparable to other chronic diseases such as diabetes and chronic obstructive lung disease.[4] Based on an analysis of a large US claims database between 2004 and 2008, direct costs due to laryngeal disorders were estimated to be between $577.18 and $953.21 per person per year.[6]

When dysphonia does not resolve in 4 weeks, further visualization and evaluation of the larynx is warranted with laryngoscopy[2] and follow-up with a multidisciplinary team including an otolaryngologist, speech therapist, and vocal pedagogue may be necessary. More studies and advances in voice therapy are needed to best identify and treat vocal cord disorders.

ANATOMY

The larynx is a cartilaginous structure with the associated muscles and ligaments in the anterior neck, which protects the lower respiratory tract from aspiration and is involved in phonation. The thyroid and cricoid cartilages form the supporting structure, and the epiglottis covers and protects the trachea during swallowing. The paired arytenoid, corniculate, and cuneiform cartilages form the support for the vocal folds or cords. The vocal folds are composed of the superior, or false, vocal folds, which do not contain muscle, and the inferior, or true vocal folds, which do contain a muscular element and are able to oppose each other (**Fig. 1**). In contrast to the rest of the respiratory tract, the vocal folds are covered by squamous epithelium instead of ciliated columnar epithelium.[7]

Innervation of the larynx is via the inferior, or recurrent, laryngeal nerve, and superior laryngeal nerve. The superior laryngeal nerve arises from the vagus nerve at the inferior ganglion and innervates the cricothyroid muscle via its external laryngeal branch.

The inferior recurrent nerves are asymmetric, with the left arising from the vagus nerve in the thorax, then looping under the aortic arch before passing superiorly to enter the larynx. The right inferior, or recurrent, laryngeal nerve arises from the vagus nerve in the neck, loops under the subclavian artery then rises superiorly to enter the larynx (**Fig. 2**). The recurrent nerves innervate the intrinsic muscles of the larynx, except the cricothyroid muscle.[7]

The intrinsic laryngeal muscles have different functions in modulating the vocal folds. The cricothyroid muscle elongates the vocal folds, leading to higher pitch. The posterior cricoarytenoid muscles cause abduction, or opening, of the vocal folds. The lateral, or anterior, cricoarytenoid muscles cause adduction, or closing of the vocal folds. The thyroarytenoid muscles relax and approximate the vocal folds. The aryepiglottic muscles adduct the aryepiglottic folds. The arytenoid muscles adduct the vocal folds.

The extrinsic muscles cause movement of the larynx and are innervated by cervical nerves and various branches of the vagus nerve and pharyngeal nerves.[7]

HISTORY/PHYSICAL EXAMINATION

A thorough history is essential to identify individuals with dysphonia that need expedited evaluation with laryngoscopy and urgent specialist referral. Complaints about

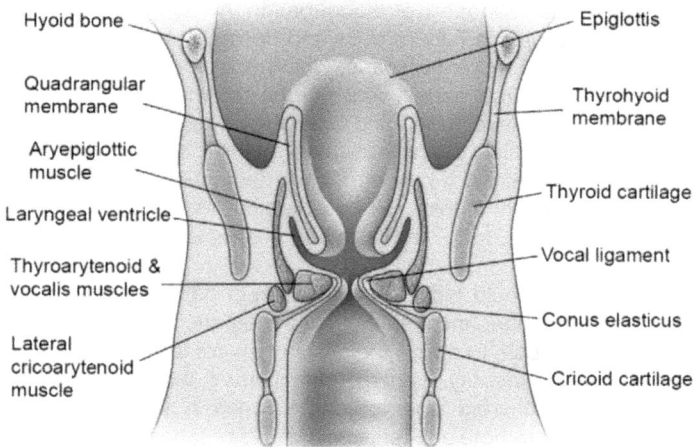

Fig. 1. Anatomy of the larynx. (*With permission from* The University of North Carolina Chapel Hill Eshelman School of Pharmacy.)

the quality of voice range from roughness, decreased range, pitch instability, and early fatigue. History includes duration, course, exact nature of concern, and associated symptoms such as anterior cervical discomfort, use of substances and medications, medical conditions including esophageal reflux, recent surgeries, and procedures,

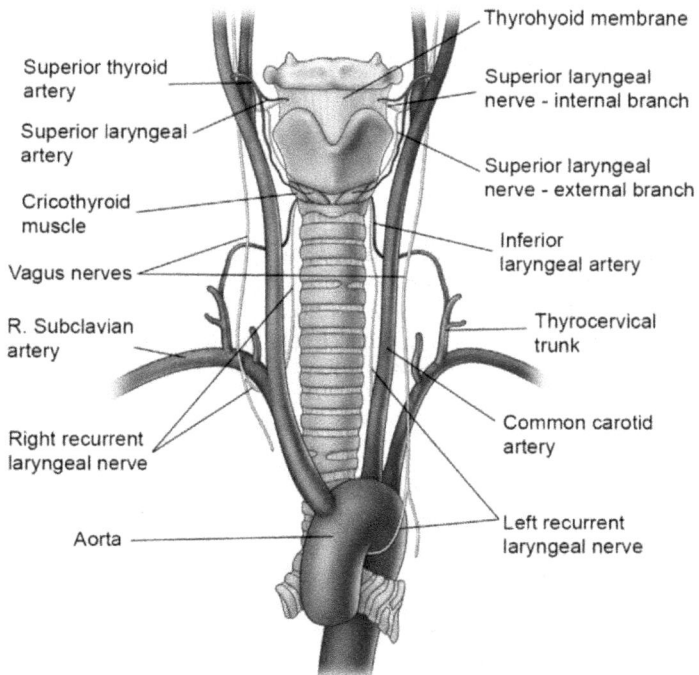

Fig. 2. Nerves and vasculature of the larynx. (*With permission from* The University of North Carolina Chapel Hill Eshelman School of Pharmacy.)

particularly endotracheal intubation, and occupation. An acute onset associated with a viral syndrome will resolve in 7 to 10 days and does not require further workup.[4]

Other etiologies include thyroid disease, which is associated with muffling of the voice, decreased range, and early vocal fatigue; pulmonary disease, which can decrease the power of air supply leading to weak voice; as well as neuromuscular disorders and posture, which can affect generation of air flow and positioning of the vocal tract. In addition, dairy products and medications that thicken mucus or decrease moisture of the vocal folds, like antihistamines, decongestants, menthols, and inhaled corticosteroids, may decrease compliance of the vocal folds leading to less vibration.[8]

Physical examination should include observation of gait and posture, noting symmetry, smoothness of motion, and weakness. As the patient speaks, note the quality, pitch, and volume of speech. Examine the oropharynx for lesions or erythema. Palpation of the neck is a key to identify overused musculature, focusing on the anterior cervical musculature, cricothyroid space, tongue base above the hyoid, and the temporomandibular joint to note any tension or areas of tenderness. Palpation should be performed both at rest and during phonation. Also palpate the thyroid and check for any lymphadenopathy. Inspect the ears and nose to ensure there is no obstruction. Respiratory examination may reveal stridor or wheezing or other findings suggestive of respiratory disease. A neurologic examination may reveal tremors, weakness, or other deficits that suggest neuromuscular disorders.[8]

Laryngoscopy should be done promptly for prolonged dysphonia, respiratory compromise, or when risk factors, particularly smoking, are present. This may require prompt referral from the primary care provider to avoid delay in diagnosis of serious conditions. Empiric therapy of dysphonia with antibiotics, anti-reflux medications, corticosteroids, and speech therapy are not recommended prior to visualization of the larynx.[4] See **Table 1** for additional recommendations for dysphonia.

DEFINITIONS
Vocal Cord Dysfunction

Often confused with asthma, individuals present with inspiratory wheezing or stridor, throat tightness, dyspnea, and anxiety related to the vocal cords paradoxically closing during inspiration.[1] Common triggers include exercise, asthma, gastroesophageal reflux, respiratory tract infections, or other irritants. Pulmonary function tests with a flattened inspiratory flow loop and nasolaryngoscopy can help diagnose vocal cord dysfunction and distinguish it from other possible etiologies. First-line therapies include therapeutic breathing maneuvers, vocal cord relaxation techniques, and treating underlying triggers.[9]

Muscle Tension Dysphonia

Dysphonia in the absence of vocal fold pathology and neurologic disorders is often caused by muscle tension dysphonia (MTD). Endoscopic visualization of the larynx, often by videostroboscopy, is crucial to the diagnosis.[10] MTD encompasses various etiologies that lead to excess paralaryngeal muscle tension. Excess tension of the extrinsic laryngeal muscles supporting the larynx leads to altered intrinsic laryngeal muscle action, causing vocal dysfunction. MTD affects primarily young to middle-aged women and includes 10% to 40% of cases seen in a voice clinic. Due to the various etiologies of MTD, treatment may include indirect voice therapy (education and vocal hygiene), direct vocal therapy, treatment of laryngeal reflux, and rarely, surgery.[10,11]

Table 1
Summary of clinical practice guideline for hoarseness (2018 American Academy of Otolaryngology-Head and Neck Surgery Foundation)

Statement	Strength of Recommendation	Rationale
1. Identification of abnormal voice Clinicians should identify dysphonia in a patient with altered voice quality, pitch, loudness, or vocal effort that impairs communication or reduces QOL.	Recommendation	Dysphonia affects quality of life and may be a symptom of underlying disease. Patient's reported symptoms, as well as proxies' collateral input should be sought.
2. Identifying underlying cause of dysphonia Clinicians should assess the patient with dysphonia by history and physical examination for underlying causes of dysphonia and factors that modify management.	Recommendation	The history of dysphonia, inciting factors, medications, and other factors should be obtained. Physical examination should focus on voice quality, head and neck examination , and respiratory evaluation.
3. Escalation of care Clinicians should assess the patient with dysphonia by history and physical examination to identify factors where expedited laryngeal evaluation is indicated. These include but are not limited to recent surgical procedures involving the head, neck, or chest; recent endotracheal intubation; presence of concomitant neck mass; respiratory distress or stridor; history of tobacco abuse; and whether the patient is a professional voice user.	Strong Recommendation	Although most dysphonia is self-limiting, the presence of risk factors such as smoking may be associated with conditions having significant morbidity and mortality. Prompt laryngoscopy may improve quality of life and outcomes.
4a. Laryngoscopy and dysphonia Clinicians may perform diagnostic laryngoscopy at any time in a patient with dysphonia.	Option	This highlights the importance of visualizing the laryngeal tissues when dysphonia is present.
4b. Need for laryngoscopy in persistent dysphonia Clinicians should perform laryngoscopy, or refer to a clinician who can perform laryngoscopy, when dysphonia fails to resolve or improve within 4 wk or irrespective of duration if a serious underlying cause is suspected.	Recommendation	Viral causes are self-limited and typically last 1–3 wk. Dysphonia of longer duration warrants laryngoscopy for diagnostic purposes.

(continued on next page)

Table 1
(continued)

Statement	Strength of Recommendation	Rationale
5. Imaging Clinicians should not obtain computed tomography (CT) or magnetic resonance imaging (MRI) for patients with a primary voice complaint prior to visualization of the larynx.	Recommendation Against	Causes of persistent dysphonia are often seen on laryngoscopy. This avoids the risks of radiation exposure with CT, side effects from MRI, and potential risks of contrast
6. Antireflux medication and dysphonia Clinicians should not prescribe antireflux medications to treat isolated dysphonia based on symptoms alone attributed to suspected gastroesophageal reflux disease (GERD) or laryngopharyngeal reflux (LPR), without visualization of the larynx.	Recommendation Against	Evidence for treating patients with dysphonia without reflux symptoms is inconclusive. Due to side effects of medications, and delay in treatment, visualization should be performed.
7. Corticosteroid therapy Clinicians should not routinely prescribe corticosteroids for patients with dysphonia prior to visualization of the larynx.	Recommendation Against	Except in limited cases, evidence does not support empiric therapy with corticosteroids, and medication has significant short- and long-term side effects.
8. Antimicrobial therapy Clinicians should not routinely prescribe antibiotics to treat dysphonia.	Strong Recommendation Against	Most acute cases of dysphonia are caused by viruses. Bacterial infections should be confirmed prior to antibiotic therapy
9a. Laryngoscopy prior to voice therapy Clinicians should perform diagnostic laryngoscopy or refer to a clinician who can perform diagnostic laryngoscopy, before prescribing voice therapy and document/communicate the results to the speech-language pathologist (SLP).	Recommendation	Laryngoscopy is necessary to establish a diagnosis and to allow appropriate therapy
9b. Advocating for voice therapy Clinicians should advocate voice therapy for patients with dysphonia from a cause amenable to voice therapy.	Strong Recommendation	Voice therapy is one of several treatments for dysphonia. Conditions such as muscle tension dysphonia, spasmodic dysphonia and Parkinson's disease may particularly benefit.

10. Surgery Clinicians should advocate for surgery as a therapeutic option for patients with dysphonia with conditions amenable to surgical intervention, such as suspected malignancy, symptomatic benign vocal fold lesions that do not respond to conservative management, or glottic insufficiency.	Recommendation	While nonsurgical management is preferred, surgery is the preferred treatment for certain lesions of the vocal fold
11. Botulinum toxin Clinicians should offer, or refer to a clinician who can offer, botulinum toxin injections for the treatment of dysphonia caused by spasmodic dysphonia and other types of laryngeal dystonia	Recommendation	Botulinum toxin is a preferred treatment for spasmodic dysphonia, in which increased laryngeal muscle tone causes dysphonia
12. Education/prevention Clinicians should inform patients with dysphonia about control/preventive measures.	Recommendation	Patient education about prevention and treatment of dysphonia should be offered to patients
13. Outcomes Clinicians should document resolution, improvement, or worsened symptoms of dysphonia or change in QOL among patients with dysphonia after treatment or observation.	Recommendation	The guideline emphasizes improving quality of care for patients with dysphonia. Patients should be followed until resolution of symptoms or appropriate diagnosis and management has been done.

Definitions: Strong Recommendation–benefits clearly exceed harms (or harms exceed benefits), and quality of evidence is excellent. Recommendation–benefits exceed harms (or harms exceed benefits), but quality of evidence is not as strong. Option–quality of evidence is low, or studies show equivocal benefit.

Data from Stachler RJ, Francis DO, Schwartz SR, et al. Clinical Practice Guideline: Hoarseness (Dysphonia) (Update) [published correction appears in Otolaryngol Head Neck Surg. 2018 Aug;159(2):403]. Otolaryngol Head Neck Surg. 2018;158(1_suppl):S1-S42. https://doi.org/10.1177/0194599817751030.

Medication-Associated Dysphonia

Medications are frequently associated with dysphonia and a thorough medication history is necessary. Antihistamines and medications with strong anticholinergic effects are commonly implicated due to their effects in drying out the mucosa. Inhaled corticosteroids predispose to mucosal irritation and fungal overgrowth. Antipsychotic medications directly cause laryngeal dystonia. Angiotensin-converting enzyme inhibitors cause a dry cough due to increased bradykinin levels.[12] Chemical laryngitis has been reported with bisphosphonates and iron pills.[13] Vascular endothelium growth factor inhibitors, such as bevacizumab, have been associated with disruption of laryngeal capillaries causing dysphonia.[14]

Vocal Fold Lesions

Vocal fold masses include nodules, polyps, cysts, and carcinoma that are diagnosed by laryngoscopic examination (**Table 2**).[15] Benign vocal fold masses are typically managed conservatively and resolve with a combination of voice hygiene and speech therapy. Fibrous mature nodules and recalcitrant polyps may require surgery.

Nodules

Often referred to as singer's nodes, nodules result from chronic, repetitive phonotrauma causing swelling of the vocal fold membranes that leads to irregular vibrations and voice pitch alterations.[16] They occur more commonly in children, adolescents, and females engaged in vocally demanding professions, including singers, kindergarten teachers, daycare workers, and call center employees. Notably, speech therapy plays a pivotal role in both surgical and non-surgical interventions. A study highlighted the significance of speech therapy, noting higher recurrence rates of nodules in patients who did not undergo speech therapy compared to those who did throughout their treatment course.[17]

Polyps

Benign sessile or peduncular lesions are caused by repetitive phonotrauma and chronic irritation from gastroesophageal reflux, smoking, exposure to irritating chemicals, or vigorous respiratory activities. The primary treatment approach involves speech therapy. Surgical intervention is necessary if the lesion persists or if the patient remains dissatisfied with their vocal quality. Less common surgical options include endoscopic laser removal, steroid injections, flexible laryngostroboscopic surgery, and acupuncture. Steroid injections have shown a 59% remission rate and a 32% improvement rate. Flexible laryngostroboscopic surgery has demonstrated success, particularly in patients with contraindications to general anesthesia or who are able to tolerate nasal fibroscopy. A study conducted in China revealed improved vocal function and reduced size of phonotraumatic lesions with acupuncture, though speech therapy treatment was deemed crucial for maintaining these improvements.[18]

Vocal cysts

These benign sac-like masses arise on the surface of vocal folds and are sometimes mistaken for nodules. Mucus retention cysts form when mucus gland ducts become obstructed, often triggered by acute respiratory infections or gastroesophageal reflux. These cysts are more prevalent in adults, particularly those working in vocally demanding fields.[19] Epidermoid cysts, resembling pearls with caseous content, develop within the subepithelial layers of vocal folds.[15] They are caused by vocal abuse or trapped epithelium within the lamina propria. Patients with cysts commonly present with symptoms of dysphonia.[19]

Table 2
Vocal fold lesions

Structure	Location	Appearance	Composition	Cause	Symptoms
Nodules	Anterior, middle 1/3 Bilateral	Callus or wart like growth Symmetric	Thickened, fibrous tissue	Repeated trauma, irritation, vocal abuse (excessive yelling, singing)	Hoarseness Rough, raspy voice quality Voice fatigue
Polyps	Unilateral, on the edge of vocal fold	Sessile, pedunculated	Fluid filled or gelatinous	Vocal misuse, yelling, speaking loudly	Hoarseness Reduced vocal endurance Sensation of lump in throat
Cysts	Unilateral, anywhere on vocal fold	Round, oval shaped lesions	Fluid or mucous-like substance on epithelial tissue	Vocal misuse, chronic irritation, present from birth	Hoarseness Vocal discomfort Sensation of lump in throat
Masses	Unilateral or Bilateral	Irregular growth, ulcerations, or thickened areas	Cancerous cells that can metastasize	Chronic irritants like smoke, alcohol, HPV, genetics	Persistent hoarseness Dysphagia Unintentional weight loss Ear pain

Data from Altman KW. Vocal Fold Masses. Otol Clin of North America. 2007;40(5):1091-1108. doi:https://doi.org/10.1016/j.otc.2007.05.011 and Schultz P. Vocal fold cancer. Eur Ann of Otorhinolaryngology, Head and Neck Diseases. 2011;128(6):301-308.

Vocal cord carcinoma

Approximately 90% of vocal cord malignancies are squamous cell carcinoma.[20] This predominantly affects males, with chronic smoking being a major risk factor and alcohol to a lesser degree.[21] Other contributing factors include human papilloma virus, herpes simplex virus, and gastroesophageal reflux. Vocal fold carcinomas present with intermittent dysphonia, which worsen with local invasion. Advanced stages of carcinoma may lead to dyspnea. Diagnosis of vocal cord carcinoma involves flexible endoscopy, with additional imaging modalities needed to assess for metastasis. These may include cervicothoracic computed tomography (CT) scans to assess vocal fold approximation and length, and thoracic CT and PET CT scans for further metastatic disease evaluation.[20]

The treatment of vocal fold carcinoma necessitates a multidisciplinary approach and depends on staging. See **Table 3** for staging. Surgical intervention for patients with T1 tumors aims to preserve the hyoid bone, cricoid cartilage, and at least 1 arytenoid cartilage, with neck dissection generally not recommended. Radiation therapy is indicated for T1 and small T2 tumors, while total laryngectomy is reserved for patients with T3 or T4 glottic tumors or T2 tumors with subglottic extension. Chemotherapy is employed for T3 and T4 tumors with positive resection margins or in cases of metastatic extracapsular adenopathy extension.[20] Recent studies have found comparable outcomes between endoscopic surgery and radiation therapy for T1 tumors. Advantages of laser cordectomy include lower cost and shorter hospital stays, though drawbacks include the use of general anesthesia and potential for decreased voice quality. Radiation therapy offers better vocal quality but is associated with increased costs, a sensation of dry larynx, and longer treatment duration.[21]

Neurologic Vocal Cord Disorders

Neurologic vocal cord disorders arise from dysfunctions in the central or peripheral nervous systems, which impact the muscles controlling the vocal cords. These disorders can significantly affect voice quality, breathing, and swallowing.

Spasmodic dysphonia

The most common focal dystonia affecting fluency of voice during speech is spasmodic dysphonia (SD) and occurs as abductor SD (ABSD) and adductor SD (ADSD).[22] Dysfunction starts at the level of the basal ganglia and expands to cerebellar and sensorimotor cortical regions. Patients diagnosed with SD are commonly female at 80% with onset occurring during the fourth decade. ABSD makes up to 15% of cases and involves uncontrollable opening of the vocal folds during voice tasks producing an excessively breathy and irregular voice. ADSD accounts for the majority of cases and has frequent and irregular closure of the vocal folds, producing a characteristic "strain and strangle" type voicing. A small subset of patients demonstrates a mixed SD characterized by a combination of adductor and abductor symptoms. The diagnosis is clinical, through laryngoscopic visualization of vocal cords and at times, electromyography. The management consists of botulinum toxin injections and voice therapy.[23]

Parkinson's disease

Parkinson's disease (PD) is a neurodegenerative disorder affecting dopaminergic neurons in the substantia nigra, leading to motor and non-motor symptoms, including vocal changes. PD is associated with voice disorders collectively referred to as hypokinetic dysarthria.[24] Most patients with PD present vocal symptoms of decreased vocal pitch, volume range, roughness, and vocal tremor.[23] Diagnosis requires voice symptoms in an individual with PD. Treatment includes standard PD medications

Table 3
Vocal cord carcinoma staging

Tumor	Description	Characteristics
T1	Limited to vocal folds with normal mobility	Superficial layer of vocal fold, does not invade into deeper layers or adjacent structures
T1a		T1a: One fold
T1b		T1b: Two folds
T2	Extension beyond vocal fold, confined to larynx	Beyond vocal fold into supraglottic, subglottic
		Vocal folds do not move normally
T3	Further extension beyond larynx, does not invade nearby structures	Invasion of thyroid cartilage, cricoid cartilage, tissues around larynx
		Vocal fold paralysis
T4	Locally advanced, invade nearby structures	T4a: invasion of thyroid cartilage, trachea, cervical soft tissue, subhyoid muscles, thyroid, esophagus
T4a		
T4b		T4b: prevertebral space, mediastinal structures, carotid artery

Data from American Joint Committee on Cancer. Oropharynx (p16-) and Hypopharynx. In: AJCC Cancer Staging Manual. 8th ed. New York, NY: Springer; 2017:123-135. 2017 American Joint Committee on Cancer.

such as carbidopa/levodopa and speech therapy techniques like Lee Silverman Voice Treatment, which is specifically designed for patients with PD to enhance the vocal volume and clarity.[25]

Unilateral true vocal cord paralysis
Immobility of 1 vocal fold is commonly related to injury of the recurrent laryngeal nerve. This results from surgical trauma, including thyroidectomy, lung tumors or neoplasms, central nervous system dysfunction, radiation, inflammation, cardiovascular disease, or idiopathic causes. Other etiologies such as systemic lupus, sarcoidosis, and tuberculosis can cause adductor vocal cord paralysis. Diagnosis requires both laryngoscopy and laryngeal electromyography of the thyroarytenoid muscle. Preferred management is monitoring for self-resolution, but voice therapy can be used as well.[23]

Bilateral abductor true vocal fold paralysis
Etiologies of vocal fold paralysis are like unilateral vocal cord paralysis. It is potentially life threatening if the folds are fixed nearly closed with associated inspiratory stridor. Presentation varies from normal phonation to complete aphonia. If there is no airway obstruction, expectant management is possible, but the presence of obstruction may require tracheostomy.[23]

Amyotrophic lateral sclerosis
Amytrophic lateral sclerosis (ALS) is a devastating disease characterized by progressive loss of both upper and lower motor neurons at the spinal or bulbar level. People with bulbar-onset ALS demonstrate various speech symptoms at the time of diagnosis, ranging from normal speech to slow, slurred speech. Individuals with slow, slurred speech should be referred for full neurologic evaluation to avoid delay in ALS diagnosis.[9] Although management options are limited, Riluzole is the first medication approved for treatment of ALS.[23]

Multiple sclerosis
Multiple sclerosis is an autoimmune demyelination disease of the central nervous system. Speech, voice, and swallowing disorders occur less frequently and occur later in the disease when the laryngeal muscles are affected. Speech disorders include abnormally long pauses between words or individual syllables of words, and slurred or hypernasal speech.[23] Treatments include immunomodulators and other chemotherapeutic agents.

Myasthenia gravis (MG)
Myasthenia gravis (MG) is an autoimmune disorder that leads to a reduction of acetylcholine in the peripheral nervous system resulting in decreased muscle contraction. With prolonged use, the intrinsic laryngeal muscles weaken, resulting in dysphonia characterized by weak and breathy voice. Recovery of voice strength with rest suggests the possibility of MG. Anticholinesterase agents such as neostigmine and pyridostigmine, thymectomy, and plasmapheresis improve symptoms.[23]

DISCUSSION

Vocal cord disorders cause significant morbidity and decreased quality-of-life. Primary care physicians have an important role in evaluating patients. However, due to risk of delayed diagnosis, prompt referral for direct laryngoscopy and advanced therapy is recommended over empiric treatment.

Further areas of study and improvement include enhancing the training of family medicine and primary care physicians in performing laryngoscopies. This may reduce delays in diagnosing serious underlying conditions requiring prompt treatment, such as malignancies.

The increased availability of point-of-care ultrasound is another avenue to diagnose vocal cord mobility problems in the primary care office setting. A meta-analysis of pediatric studies demonstrates a sensitivity of 91% and a specificity of 97% to detect vocal cord immobility.[26] In adults, a systematic review showed a sensitivity of 95% and a specificity of 99%.[27]

SUMMARY

Vocal cord disorders consist of a variety of conditions that range from mild dysphonia to airway obstruction (bilateral true focal cord paralysis). Etiologies range from idiopathic vocal cord dysfunction to medication induced dysphonia, anatomic masses, and neurologic disorders.

History, physical examination, and often laryngoscopy are necessary to arrive at a definitive diagnosis. A combination of duration of symptoms, risk factors, voice quality, fatigue, and associated symptoms are important to suggest diagnosis. Laryngoscopy is a supportive diagnostic test that helps identify vocal cord function. Vocal fold masses often lead to vocal cord dysfunction, with most being benign, though a minority may be malignant. Nodules, polyps, and cysts can exhibit similar clinical features but can be discerned through direct visualization. Initial treatment includes a combination of voice hygiene and speech therapy. Voice hygiene may include a period of complete voice silence for 1 week. Maintaining hydration is crucial and use of a humidifier can assist to keep the vocal cords moist for optimal vibration. Avoid common medications that may dry or irritate the vocal folds including inhaled corticosteroids, antihistamines, decongestants, topical analgesics, and mentholated preparations.[28] Typically, these structural anomalies improve with speech therapy trials, but if no progress is seen, surgical intervention along with continued speech therapy are necessary. For vocal cord masses, recommendations include quitting smoking, undergoing speech therapy, and maintaining close surveillance. For neurologic disorders, treatment varies from botulinum toxin injections to voice therapy and medications that treat the underlying neurologic disease.

CLINICS CARE POINTS

- Several key evidence-based statements from the AAO-HNSF in the diagnosis and treatment of dysphonia include the following:
  - Prompt laryngeal evaluation should be prompted by risk factors, such as recent surgical procedures of the head and neck region; recent endotracheal intubation; respiratory compromise; tobacco use; and professional voice user.
  - Laryngoscopy should be performed when dysphonia persists for more than 4 w or in the presence of risk factors.
  - Visualization of the larynx for dysphonia should be done prior to MRI or CT, prescribing anti-reflux medications for suspected gastroesophageal reflux, prescribing corticosteroids, or referral to voice therapy.
  - Antibiotics should not be routinely prescribed to treat dysphonia.[4]
- Nodules, polyps, and cysts are common benign masses, which cause vocal cord dysfunction due to repetitive vocal cord use.
- While there are differing opinions on the treatment options for benign lesions, all sources recommend speech therapy as either primary treatment or in combination with surgical removal.

DISCLOSURES

None of the authors have any disclosures.

REFERENCES

1. Malaty J, Wu V. Vocal cord dysfunction: rapid evidence review. AFP 2021;104(5): 471–5.
2. Neighbors C, Hashmi MF, Song SA. Dysphonia. In: StatPearls. Treasure Island (FL): StatPearls Publishing; 2024.
3. Hong I, Bae S, Lee HK, et al. Prevalence of dysphonia and dysphagia among adults in the United States in 2012 and 2022. Am J Speech Lang Pathol 2024.
4. Stachler RJ, Francis DO, Schwartz SR, et al. Clinical practice guideline: hoarseness (dysphonia) (update). Otolaryngol Head Neck Surg 2018;158(1_suppl): S1–42 [published correction appears in Otolaryngol Head Neck Surg 2018;159(2):403].
5. Cohen SM, Kim J, Roy N, et al. The impact of laryngeal disorders on work-related dysfunction. Laryngoscope 2012;122(7):1589–94. Epub 2012 May 1. PMID: 22549455.
6. Cohen SM, Kim J, Roy N, et al. Direct health care costs of laryngeal diseases and disorders. Laryngoscope 2012;122(7):1582–8.
7. Suárez-Quintanilla J, Fernández Cabrera A, Sharma S. Anatomy, head and neck: larynx. In: StatPearls [internet]. Treasure Island (FL): StatPearls Publishing; 2024.
8. Naunheim MR, Fink DS, Courey MS. The professional voice. In: Cummings CW, Haughey H, Regan T, et al, editors. Cummings Otolaryngology: head and neck surgery. 7th edition. Philadelphia, PA: Elsevier Mosby Publisher; 2020. p. 839–56.
9. Vieira H, Costa N, Sousa T, et al. Voice-based classification of amyotrophic lateral sclerosis: where are we and where are we going? A systematic review. Neurodegener Dis 2019;19(5–6):163–70.
10. Ferrán S, Garaycochea O, Terrasa D, et al. Biography of muscle tension dysphonia: a scoping review. Appl Sci 2024;14(5):2030.
11. Van Houtte E, Van Lierde K, Claeys S. Pathophysiology and treatment of muscle tension dysphonia: a review of the current knowledge. J Voice 2011;25(2):202–7.
12. Schwartz SR, Cohen SM, Dailey SH, et al. Clinical practice guideline: hoarseness (dysphonia). Otolaryngol Head Neck Surg 2009;141(3 Suppl 2):S1–31.
13. Sethia R, Bishop R, Gordian-Arroyo A, et al. Iron pill-induced chemical laryngitis. Ann Otol Rhinol Laryngol 2023;132(1):91–4.
14. Carter CA, Caroen SZ, Oronsky AL, et al. Dysphonia after bevacizumab rechallenge: a case report. Case Rep Oncol 2015;8(3):423–5.
15. Altman KW. Vocal Fold masses. Otolaryngol Clin 2007;40(5):1091–108.
16. Wallis L, Jackson-Menaldi C, Holland W, et al. Vocal fold nodule vs. vocal fold polyp: answer from surgical pathologist and voice pathologist point of view. J Voice 2004;18(1):125–9.
17. Cohen SM, Garrett CG. Utility of voice therapy in the management of vocal fold polyps and cysts. Otolaryngol Head Neck Surg 2007;136(5):742–6.
18. Vasconcelos D, Gomes A, Araújo C. Vocal Fold polyps: literature review. Int Arch Otorhinolaryngol 2019;23(01):116–24.
19. Martins RHG, Santana MF, Tavares ELM. Vocal cysts: clinical, endoscopic, and surgical aspects. J Voice 2011;25(1):107–10.
20. Schultz P. Vocal fold cancer. Eur Ann Otorhinolaryngol Head Neck Dis 2011; 128(6):301–8.

21. Amornmarn R, Prempree T, Viravathana T, et al. A therapeutic approach to early vocal cord carcinoma. Acta Radiol Oncol 2009;24(4):321–5.
22. Mor N, Simonyan K, Blitzer A. Central voice production and pathophysiology of spasmodic dysphonia. Laryngoscope 2018;128(1):177–83.
23. Sapienza C, Hoffman B, Voice disorders, 4th edition, 2022, Plural Publishing, Inc; San Diego. Available at: https://www.pluralpublishing.com/publications/voice-disorders-1. (Accessed 13 June 2024).
24. Kovac D, Mekyska J, Galaz Z, et al. 2021. Multilingual analysis of speech and voice disorders in patients with Parkinson's disease. 2021 44th international conference on telecommunications and signal processing (TSP), 26-28 July 2021, Brno, Czech Republic, https://doi.org/10.1109/TSP52935.2021.9522597.
25. Pu T, Huang M, Kong X, et al. Lee silverman voice treatment to improve speech in Parkinson's disease: a systemic review and meta-analysis. Parkinsons Dis 2021; 27:3366870.
26. Hamilton CE, Su E, Tawfik D, et al. Assessment of vocal cord motion using laryngeal ultrasound in children: a systematic review and meta-analysis. Pediatr Crit Care Med 2021;22(10):e532–9.
27. Su E, Hamilton C, Tawfik DS, et al. Laryngeal ultrasound detects Vocal Fold immobility in adults: a systematic review. J Ultrasound Med 2022;41(8):1873–88.
28. Weston Z, Schneider SL. Demystifying vocal hygiene: considerations for professional voice users. Curr Otorhinolaryngology Reports 2023;11:387–94.

Head and Neck Cancers

Archana Kudrimoti, MBBS, MPH[a],*, Mahesh R. Kudrimoti, MD[b]

KEYWORDS

- Head and neck cancer • Human papilloma virus • Multidisciplinary teams

KEY POINTS

- Head neck cancers are heterogenous cancers with rising incidence of treatable/curative cancers.
- Human papilloma virus and tobacco use are major risk factors.
- They are treated comprehensively by multidisciplinary teams involving surgery, radiation, chemotherapy, and ancillary services.
- With rising survival in certain subsets, it is important for primary care providers to be aware of long-term surveillance and sequela.

INTRODUCTION

Head and neck cancers are cancers that arise in the mucosa and spread to the lymph nodes in the neck and can metastasize to other areas in the body such as lung, liver, and bone. They constitute 4% of all cancers in the United States of America (USA) and are the seventh leading cause of cancer worldwide.[1] These cancers can arise in the oral cavity, oropharynx, larynx, pharynx, sinus areas, and nasopharynx. Non-mucosal cancers of the head and neck can also arise in the parotid glands and other endocrine glands such as thyroid. We will limit our discussion to the cancers that arise predominantly from the mucosal lining of the head and neck area.

The sites and subsites from which these cancers can arise dictate the management decisions. It is important to understand the anatomy and pattern of lymphatic spread of each subsite as there is a considerable variation within each subsite. The definition of each site is as follows (**Fig. 1**):[2]

Oral cavity: Oral cavity includes the lips, the anterior two-thirds of the tongue, the mucosa of the cheek (buccal mucosa) and lips, the floor of mouth, hard palate, and retromolar trigone.

[a] Department of Family and Community Medicine, University of Kentucky, UK Healthcare at Turfland, 2195 Harrodsburg Road, Suite 125, Lexington, KY 40504, USA; [b] St Elizabeth Cancer Center, 17525 Greendale Plaza Drive, Greendale, IN 47025, USA
* Corresponding author.
E-mail address: Akudr2@email.uky.edu

Prim Care Clin Office Pract 52 (2025) 139–155
https://doi.org/10.1016/j.pop.2024.09.014   **primarycare.theclinics.com**
0095-4543/25/© 2024 Elsevier Inc. All rights reserved, including those for text and data mining, AI training, and similar technologies.

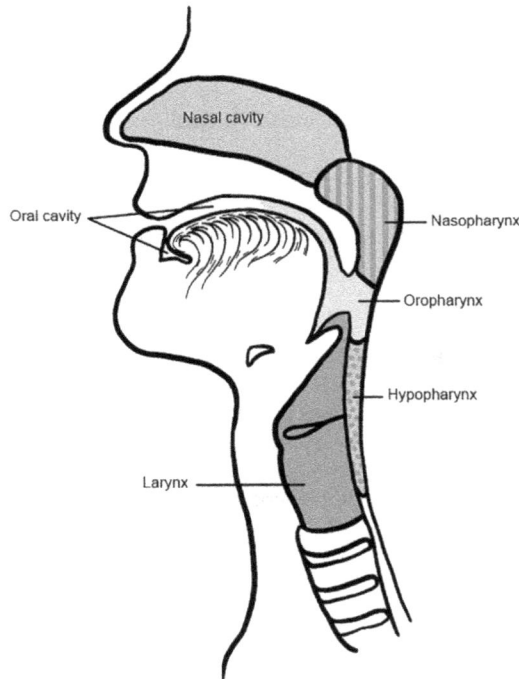

Fig. 1. Anatomy of head and neck.

Oropharynx: The oropharynx includes the soft palate, the tonsils and the tonsillar pillars, and the base of tongue (posterior third of the tongue). The incidence of human papillomavirus (HPV) positive tumors is highest in this subsite.

Nasopharynx: Nasopharynx is the part behind the nasal cavity and superior to the soft palate. The Eustachian tube opens on the lateral walls. It has rich lymphatics, and the incidence of lymph nodal spread is over 70% at presentation. The cancers in this subsite are related to Epstein-Barr virus (EBV) infection and common in South Asia. It is more frequently seen in the coastal areas of the USA. These cancers are mostly managed non-surgically.

Hypopharynx: Hypopharynx is the area extending from the posterior larynx to esophageal opening. It includes the pyriform sinus, posterior pharyngeal wall, and post cricoid area. Cancers in this area are uncommon and present with dysphagia and invasion into larynx or lateral neck.

Larynx: Larynx comprises the voice box with subsites including the supraglottic, glottic, and subglottic tumors. Tumors of the glottis have limited lymphatic spread in contrast to the other sites and tend to present earlier than other subsites. Subglottic tumors are uncommon in presentation.

Nasal Cavity and Paranasal sinuses: Tumors of these areas tend to invade locally with involvement of skull base and orbital invasion.

EPIDEMIOLOGY

It is estimated by the American Cancer Society, that there will be close to 66,920 cases of oral cavity and pharyngeal cancers diagnosed in the USA and there will be approximately 15,400 deaths from disease progression.[3] In the USA, the incidence of HPV associated oropharyngeal cancers is increasing and there is a drop in the incidence of non-HPV related cancers. Over 75% of current oropharyngeal cancers are related to HPV infection. HPV can be detected in cancers of other sites in the head and neck, but it does not impact management decisions to the same extent.[4] EBV virus infection is the common etiologic factor for nasopharyngeal cancers.[5,6] Radiation exposure and some genetic diseases such as Fanconi anemia are associated with higher risk of head and neck cancers. Chewing betel nut is implicated as a causative agent in buccal mucosa cancers on the Indian subcontinent.

BURDEN OF DISEASE

The incidence of these cancers has shown a 1% increase per year over the past 2 decades. This reflects the increase in the rise of the HPV-associated oropharyngeal cancers. These are more in the 40 to 50 y old population and non-smokers and are related to HPV exposure. It is increasingly recognized that these are biologically different from the non-HPV associated cancers and have a different outcome and clinical behavior.[4,7] The management of these cancers has been changing with better identification of prognostic factors and higher anticipated survival. Survivors of head and neck cancers often deal with the sequalae of therapy as they are living longer, it is anticipated that the primary care physicians are going to encounter more patients in their clinics in the coming years.[1,2]

PATHOGENESIS

Most head and neck cancers arise from the mucosa of the head and neck. More than 90% of these are squamous cell cancers and other cancers such as lymphomas, sarcomas, and adenocarcinomas can arise from these areas but the management for those cancers is different and will not be discussed in this article. The known risk factors for these cancers are the use of tobacco products in any form, as well as alcohol consumption.[8] The risk is increased 30-fold or so in people who smoke and drink heavily.[9–12] Other contributory factors in non-smokers is the HPV-associated cancers transmitted through sexual contact. There is robust evidence of causation of nasopharyngeal cancers and EBV infection especially from Southeast Asia.[5,6]

CLINICAL PRESENTATION

Most head and neck cancers present with symptoms from where they arise (**Table 1**)[13] (**Fig. 2**).[14]

There are close to 300 to 400 lymph nodes in the head and neck area and involvement of lymph nodes is common at presentation. Based on the location of the primary site the involvement of lymph nodes may vary. The incidence of lymph nodal spread is higher amongst the tongue and floor of mouth cancers in contrast to other subsites. Base of tongue cancers tend to present with adenopathy in the neck and often asymptomatic primary tumors. The sinus and oral cavity cancers as a rule tend to have less than 5% incidence of lymph node involvement whereas lymph nodal enlargement in the neck may be a presenting sign for a cancer arising from the oropharynx or laryngeal areas.

About 2% to 5% of tumors that present with lymph node enlargement in the neck are without an obvious primary site. These are thought to arise from an unknown (occult) primary site. The cancers that behave in this fashion usually arise from the tonsil, base of tongue, nasopharynx, or the pyriform sinus areas. Bilateral nodal

Table 1
Most common symptoms based on anatomic site

Oral Cavity	Nasal Cavity	Pharynx	Larynx
Non-healing ulcers in mouth	Epistaxis	Nasopharynx - cranial nerve involvement, orbital and visual changes massive LNE	Changes in voice hoarseness
Leucoplakia or Erythroplakia	Nasal blockage -unilateral	Oropharynx - LNE, dysphagia, odynophagia, tonsillitis, referred pain to ear	Swallowing choking spells
Pain at the site or referred pain to ear- late stage	Anosmia	Hypopharynx- mostly silent and present with LNE. late stage - dysphagia and weight loss	Late stage-stridor referred pain to ear
Lump/Lymph node enlargement (LNE)			Weight loss
Dysphagia, choking on food weight loss- late stage			

Table was generated by author based on review of published literature.

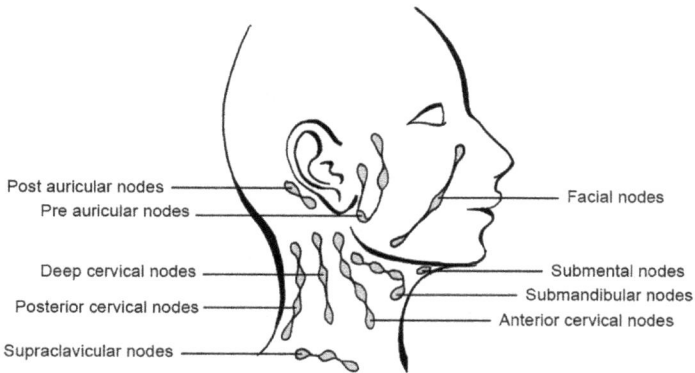

Fig. 2. Lymphatic system of head and neck.

involvement is common in tumors arising from the nasopharynx (40%), base of tongue (40%), supraglottic laryngeal cancers (15%), and soft palate cancers (15%). It is less common (10%) with tonsillar cancers, hypopharyngeal cancers, and oral tongue. Glottic tumors rarely have lymph nodal spread unless the tumors have spread into other subsites in the larynx. Lip and subglottic tumors have low lymph nodal involvement overall.[13]

CANCER MANAGEMENT

Cancer management of mucosal tumors is based on tissue pathology, stage of cancer, and co-morbid factors. All cancers are staged based on information obtained from imaging modalities and clinical examinations. The staging is clinical if patients do not undergo surgery and categorized as pathologic if patients are resected and have a lymph nodal dissection performed.

Non-mucosal cancers: The other common non-mucosal cancers in the head and neck area tend to arise from the salivary glands or as lymph nodal deposits from skin of the face. They tend to be unilateral and treated with surgery and assessed for adjuvant therapy based on risk factors. The major salivary glands are the parotids (majority of cases), submandibular, and submental glands. The minor salivary glands are distributed on the hard and soft palate and other areas in the nasopharynx and oropharynx. The incidence of these cancers is extremely low, probably less than 5%. Parotids tend to be a site of metastatic disease from skin cancers. Primary squamous cell cancers of the parotid are extremely rare, and most are lymph nodes metastasize from the skin of the face (**Box 1**).[15,16]

Initial assessment of the primary site and lymph nodes can be made based on a contrast computed tomography (CT) scan of the head and neck including the skull bases and the thoracic inlet. For hypopharyngeal tumors, the scan should include the carina if a concomitant CT chest is not being performed. Imaging of the chest can be with or without contrast, but most patients have CT scans of the neck and chest performed simultaneously.[17] An alternate imaging modality to characterize the primary site is an MRI with contrast. CT scans can be useful in situations where MRI is deficient including cortical bone, periosteal or cartilage involvement, or destruction. MRI is recommended when patients have dental fillings that impede and artifact CT images, suspect marrow invasion, cranial nerve involvement and perineural spread, orbital and skull base spread through the foramina, and for differentiating mucus plugs from

---

Box 1
Tests for diagnosis and treatment planning

- Detailed medical history and complete physical including head and neck examination including screening for Depression.
- Mirror and Fiberoptic examination if needed.
- Endoscopy and examination under anesthesia (EUA)as needed.
- Biopsy of tumor or Lymph node site - HPV testing by p16 for throat cancers and EBV (DNA) for nasopharynx- Fine needle aspiration cytology of Lymph Node or tissue biopsy-special stains for genetic analysis for immunotherapy.
- CT with contrast and/or MRI with and without contrast of primary tumor and neck-include skull bases and thoracic inlet.
- CT chest with or without contrast.
- Imaging for distant metastasis – FDG-PET/CT.
- Dental Examination with Panorex.
- Nutrition, speech, and swallow evaluation.
- Hearing test.
- Eye and endocrine evaluation for nasopharyngeal cancer.
- Smoking cessation counseling.
- Screening for Hepatitis B.

Box was generated by author based on review of published literature.

---

tumor, especially in the sinuses. Ultrasound of the neck is useful in establishing tissue diagnosis and in follow-up. Panoramic X-rays are recommended for dental evaluation and extractions. PET scan is done for establishing the metabolic activity at the initiation of therapy and for assessing response 3 months post completion of all therapy. It has prognostic value and a negative PET scan at 3 months is a positive predictor of complete response and favorable outcome.[18,19] Most patients will not need additional metabolic imaging after a negative PET scan and can be followed with CT/MRI/ultrasound sonography test as indicated. CT/MRI/PET scans are useful in surgical and radiation planning with use of these modalities for fusion studies and dose prescription (**Table 2**).

GOALS AND PRINCIPLES OF TREATMENT

Unlike other cancers, such as lung or pancreatic cancer, head, and neck cancers tend to remain confined to the neck and do not rapidly metastasize to other parts of the body. Most cancers tend to fail locally at the site of origin or the lymph nodes in the neck. Widespread metastatic disease to the lung and bones at diagnosis is uncommon and sign of the advanced stage. Multiplicity of lymph nodal involvement increases the odds of metastatic disease. It is of paramount importance to control disease at the primary site and in the lymph nodal chain/group. The use of surgery or radiation as the primary treatment is based on the location of the primary, organ function, resectability, pattern of lymph nodal involvement, extent of reconstruction needed, and patient preference. Most cases need multi-modal management involving the use of surgery, radiation, and chemotherapy.[1,20,21] It is common for patients to need alternate avenues for nutrition and breathing conduits, such as feeding tubes

Table 2
Staging comparisons of Head Neck cancer subsites per American Joint Committee on cancer (AJCC)

Tumor	Oral Cancer	Oropharyngeal HPV +	Nasopharynx (NP)	Oropharyngeal HPV-Hypopharynx	Larynx
T1	<2 cm <5 mm DOI	<2 cm	Confined to NP, Nasal cavity	<2 cm	1 subsite, Vocal cord
T2	<2 to <4 cm DOI >5 mm to ≤ 10 mm	2–4 cm	Parapharyngeal extension	2–4 cm	>2 subsites
T3	>4 cm	>4 cm	Invasion into Skull base, PNS	>4 cm	Limited to larynx with fixation of vocal cords, paraglottic spread or erosion of thyroid cartilage
T4a	Invades cortical bone, skin, nerves, extrinsic muscles of tongue muscle	Invades laryngeal surface of epiglottis	Intracranial extension, involvement of cranial nerves, orbit, hypopharynx, infratemporal space/ masticator space	Invades Larynx, extrinsic tongue muscles, medial pterygoids, hard palate or mandible	Invades beyond larynx into trachea, soft tissue neck, strap muscles, extrinsic tongue muscles, thyroid, esophagus or through Thyroid cartilage
T4b	Invasion into masticator space, Pterygoid plates, skull base or Internal carotid artery	Invasion into Larynx, extrinsic tongue muscles, hard palate, mandible, medial Pterygoid		Invasion into Lateral Pterygoid, pterygoid plates skull base, lateral nasopharynx or encases carotid artery	Prevertebral space, Encases carotid artery, mediastinal structures

Node	Oral Cancer	Oropharyngeal	Nasopharynx	Oropharyngeal HPV-Hypopharynx	Larynx
N0	No LN	No LN	No LN	No LN	No LN
N1	Single LN <3 cm, ENE neg	Single <6 cm	Unilateral 6 cm above cricoid cartilage, Uni or Bil retropharyngeal LN <6 cm	<3 cm No ENE	<3 cm No ENE
N2a	>3 cm to <6 cm ENE Neg	Bilateral or Contralateral <6 cm	Bilateral <6 cm above cricoid	Same as OC	Same as OC
N2b	>2 nodes none >6 cm size	NA	NA	Same as OC	Same as OC

(continued on next page)

Table 2
(continued)

Node	Oral Cancer	Oropharyngeal	Nasopharynx	Oropharyngeal HPV-Hypopharynx	Larynx
N2c	Bilateral <6 cm size	NA	NA	Same as OC	
N3a	>6 cm ENE Neg	>6 cm in size	>6 cm below cricoid		
N3b	>6 cm ENE (+)				

Table was generated by author based on review of published literature.

Abbreviations: ENE, extra nodal extension; LN, lymph nodes; N, node; OC, oral cavity; PNS, paranasal sinusus; T, tumor.

and tracheostomies. In some cases, such as advanced oral cavity cancers or laryngeal cancers, the patients may have permanent feeding tubes or tracheostomies. Use of feeding tubes is also common during chemoradiation therapy.

Surgery

The goal of surgery in head and neck cancer is to resect the primary site with clear margins preserve function of the organ to the best of its ability. Margin status is of paramount importance in reducing local recurrence and addition of dose escalation of radiation therapy and chemotherapy. Frozen sections are often used during surgery to ascertain complete clearance of the tumor but the final decision for adjuvant therapy depends on the final stained pathology specimen. A good rule of the thumb for clear surgical margins is clearance beyond 1 to 1.5 cm for the gross tumor. Smaller margins are acceptable in situations such as the larynx where extensive resection could compromise function.[22] Based on the size of the tumor and function of the organ, surgery might entail resection of the entire organ such as an advanced larynx cancer or tongue cancer. Reconstruction with flaps and tissue grafts are an important consideration when surgery involves resection of a large volume of the primary site. Surgery often includes resection of the lymph nodes in the neck, which is either combined with the primary surgery or performed a few days later. Depending on the extent it may be selective, modified, or radical neck dissection.[23,24] The lymph nodes in the neck are dissected en bloc and assessed for risk factors. Decision for additional radiation, with or without chemotherapy, is often made based on the number of lymph nodes involved, levels of lymph nodes involved, size, and presence of extra capsular extension. Surgery is the predominant mode of management in cancers of the oral cavity, sinus cancers, and advanced larynx cancers with no option of organ preservation, hypopharyngeal cancers with poor functional options, smaller tumors of the oropharynx (less than 4 cm – using a robotic approach) and early stage base of tongue cancers (robotic approach). Transoral robotic surgery is often used in HPV-positive oropharyngeal and selected laryngeal cancers that present with small primary tumors and neck nodes. The surgical margins of less than 5 mm may be acceptable in certain cases but most need adjuvant radiation therapy. About 10% to 15% of the cases may not need adjuvant therapy based on results of clinical trials. Use of robotic surgery has allowed for reduction of multimodal cancer treatments and has allowed for radiation therapy dose de-escalation. Reduction in use of dose of radiation therapy and elimination of chemotherapy improves the quality-of-life of patients without affecting survival rates. Surgery has a limited role in the management of nasopharyngeal and early to advanced oropharyngeal and base of tongue cancers, early-stage larynx cancers with good voice and swallowing function, and early stage hypopharyngeal cancers. Surgery for sinus cancers involves extensive coordination with ear, nose, and throat, oro-maxillary, and sometimes neurosurgic or ophthalmology teams as skull base invasion or orbital invasion is seen in advanced cancers.

Radiation Therapy

Radiation therapy is extensively used in head and neck cancer as a primary treatment or as an adjuvant therapy following surgery and as a palliative modality in very advanced cancers. Majority of cancers are treated with external beam radiation therapy using linear accelerators.[25] There are some centers that perform brachytherapy for selected cases of the oral cavity and nasopharynx, but the practice has declined over a period. Radiation therapy is used for organ preservation in cancers of the nasopharynx, oropharynx, larynx (with good function), and hypopharynx (selected cases). Radiation therapy is a daily treatment for 6 to 7 weeks depending on the goals of therapy.[26–28] Based on the clinical situation, it is combined with chemotherapy delivery. The chemotherapeutic agents act as radiation sensitizers and have shown survival advantage in advanced cases compared to radiation alone. There have been significant gains in radiation oncology technology with the development of image-guided therapy, adoption of intensity modulated radiation therapy, limiting normal tissue toxicity, and side effects of therapy. Some centers have been using proton therapy for limiting acute and chronic side effects of therapy.[29,30]

Chemotherapy

Chemotherapy is used as a radiation enhancing modality in a definitive setting when patients are being treated with a goal of organ preservation, or as a palliative mode in metastatic disease. A variety of chemotherapeutic agents have been tried in the head and neck cancers. The most active agent used extensively is cisplatin either weekly or once every 3 w. It is important to identify the agent used, as toxicity profiles are different with various agents and their combination with radiation therapy.[31–33]

Immunotherapy

The role for immunomodulation of head and neck cancers was established with the recognition that cetuximab, which is an endothelial growth factor receptor inhibitor was effective in head and neck cancer when used alone or in combination with radiation. There was a 5-y survival advantage for patients treated with Cetuximab and radiation compared to radiation alone. Since then, there has been increased recognition of use of programmed cell death ligand-1 inhibitors in head and neck cancers in locally advanced or a metastatic setting or use in patients that refuse or cannot tolerate chemotherapy. It is important for primary physicians to be aware of the chronic toxicities like endocrine problems, as well as immune-mediated effects on various organs from these agents as they are often on the regimens for prolonged periods of time (weeks to months)[34,35] (**Table 3**).

PATIENT MONITORING AND SIDE EFFECTS
Supportive Care

Patients often live with side effects of combined modality treatments. It is important for the primary care physician to recognize the acute and chronic side effects of each intervention in clinical practice. Side effects can be due to multiple interventions and recognizing them can guide the primary care physician to address it with appropriate specialists.[36]

Nutritional issues - Most head and neck cancer patients have an element of malnutrition and weight loss due to the nature of the cancer and lifestyle choices and side

Table 3		
Systemic therapy agents actively used in treatment of head neck cancers		
Chemotherapy	Carboplatin	Hydoxyurea
	Capecitabine	Methotrexate
	Cisplatin	Paclitaxel
	Docetaxel	Pemetrexed
	5-Fluorouracil P	
Targeted Therapy	Afatinib	Cetuximab
Immunotherapy	Ipilimumab	Nivolumab
	Pembrolizumab	Toripalimab-tpzi

Table was generated by author based on review of published literature.

effects of multimodal management. Anchoring nutrition during treatment and rehabilitation is of paramount importance in patient well-being and recovery. Aggressive nutrition management, which is personalized to patient needs in consultation of a dietician, is encouraged in patients who have lost 5% of baseline weight in 1 mo or 10% over 6 mo; or in patients who have compromised swallowing function as a result of large primary tumor in the aerodigestive pathway. Patients receiving radiation therapy should be monitored very closely for malnutrition and weight loss. Follow-up with dietary is recommended till the patient regains baseline weight. This milestone often may take considerable time and support for the patient.[37–39]

Speech and Swallowing issues - Patients should be seen at regular intervals by the speech and swallowing team to monitor changes from baseline. Speech and swallowing exercises are often given to patients during these meetings. The follow-up period should extend till baseline improvement is noted and this may extend for a considerable amount of time. Speech rehabilitation post laryngectomy can include esophageal speech and use of an electrolarynx called Tracheoesophageal (TE) voice restoration. Electrolarynx is a battery-operated device, which mimics sounds based on vibration of the skin of the neck. TE voice restoration is used by many people after a laryngectomy. TE speech is similar to normal laryngeal speech because it uses air from the lungs to power speech production just as it did before laryngectomy. A small, removable device called a voice prosthesis, sits inside the stoma, and allows air from the lungs to pass into the esophagus for sound production. The sound then travels into the mouth for speech.

Other oral issues - Patients experience dysgeusia, xerostomia, chronic pain, trismus, lymphedema, and restriction of movements of the neck especially at the shoulders especially if a neck dissection is performed with compromise of the accessory nerve. Patients often need referral to physical therapy for rehabilitation and management of lymphedema. Early involvement of these supportive services results in better functional outcome as reversal of chronic changes such as fibrosis is often challenging.[36,37] Thrush (candidiasis) is very commonly seen in the oral cavity and topical lozenges, nystatin, or oral fluconazole/itraconazole may be used to treat the condition. These are prescribed for a minimum of 7 to 14 days. Refractory cases may need referral to infectious disease for consideration of additional agents. Trismus is a debilitating side effect of surgical and radiation therapy interventions, especially if the primary was T3 or larger and involved the retromolar trigone and the oropharyngeal area. Gentle and regular stretching exercises and use of tongue blades to sustain gains is encouraged. Patients can have custom mouth opening devices to help with stretching and improve the bite opening.

Dental care - The other aspect of chronic changes from multimodal therapy involves dental care and taste changes induced by therapeutic intervention, especially radiation therapy. Radiation therapy to the head and neck area results in reduction of salivary flow and can affect every aspect of oral cavity function. The teeth are more susceptible to caries and patient need ongoing dental care to reduce the incidence of dento-alveolar infections, and chances of osteoradionecrosis (seen in heavily irradiated patients with tumors close to the mandible especially oropharyngeal cancers). High potency topical fluoride use for the long-term is usually recommended to reduce the incidence of caries. Lack of saliva encourages bacterial overgrowth in the oral cavity and leads to caries.[40] Dental caries may be apparent within 3 months of completion of radiation therapy, especially if the patients are percutaneous endoscopic gastroenterostomy tubes (PEG)-dependent and do not perform ideal oral hygiene. Dental extractions should be done with care especially in irradiated patients as risk of poor wound healing and abscess formation post-procedure are high. Patients often require hyperbaric oxygen before and after procedures to help reduce injury and enhance recovery following extraction.[41]

Brushing and flossing at least twice a day is minimally recommended and ideally performed post each meal. Changes in lifestyle and type of diet can influence the development of these changes. Strategies to reduce xerostomia include increased fluid intake with limitations of alcohol and acidic foods. The use of salivary substitutes may help. These include gels containing lysozyme, lactoferrin peroxidase, and super-saturated calcium phosphate solutions. Some trials have shown the benefit of using salivary stimulants such as pilocarpine and cevimeline.[42–44] Stimulants such as xylitol chewing gum and sorbitol/malic acid lozenges may help symptomatically (**Table 4**).

EMERGING THERAPIES

With rising incidence of HPV related tumors, the emphasis of treatment is shifting toward de-escalation of treatment intensity and identification of patients that do not need Trimodality Therapy of surgery, radiation, and chemotherapy. Surgical techniques including wide spread use of robotic surgery, new radiation therapy modalities, such as volume modulated arc therapy, proton therapy, and identification of gene alterations for future immunotherapeutic targets are being tested in clinical trials.[45–48] Other trials are focused on reduction of the burden of disease by epidemiologic intervention such as HPV vaccination. As patients live with significant side effects of therapy, clinical trials in reducing mucositis and xerostomia are also being conducted.[49,50]

SURVIVORSHIP CARE PLAN

Effective communication at the oncology/primary care interface may allow survivors to feel they have the continuity of care they desire (**Box 2**). Depending on the stage of cancer and modalities used head and neck cancer survivors can experience a wide variety of long-term effects. The goals of survivorship plan include prevention of new and recurrent cancers and managing late effects, surveillance for cancer—recurrence or second cancers, assessment of impact of therapeutic intervention on psychosocial, physical, and immunologic effects (medical issues, symptoms, psychologic distress, and financial and social concerns). Coordination of care between primary care providers and specialists ensures that the survivor's health needs are

Table 4
Outcomes of Head Neck cancer subsites by reported 5 year survival

Site	Local (LN Negative)	Regional (LN Positive)	Metastatic (M-1 or 4 B)
Overall (all sites)	86%	69%	40%
Larynx	78%	46%	34%
Hypopharynx	61%	39%	28%
Nasopharynx	82%	72%	49%
Sinuses	86%	52%	43%
Lip	94%	63%	38%
Tongue	84%	70%	41%
Floor of the mouth	73%	42%	23%
Oropharynx	59%	62%	29%

Table was generated by author based on review of published literature.

Box 2
Cancer survivorship care plan

Medical history and physical examination including complete head and neck examination and Fiberoptic examination/indirect laryngoscopy
- Year 1, every 1 to 3 mo.
- Year 2, every 2 to 6 mo.
- Years 3 through 5 y, every 4 to 8 mo.
- Over 5 y, every 12 mo.

Blood tests to look for hormonal changes after site specific treatments—TSH q 6 to 12 mo if pre-tracheal radiation, cortisol/ACTH, LH (Base of skull radiation).

Imaging tests for recurrence and second cancers based on site of primary cancer and symptoms.

Carotid dopplers – assess for Carotid stenosis after head and neck radiation.

Ongoing assessments with standard tools for cognitive decline, chronic pain, sleep disorders, and delirium.

Dental examination and optimal dental hygiene for areas exposed to radiation.

Optimize physical activity, healthy diet, and weight management.

Supportive care, as needed
- Speech, hearing, and swallowing evaluation and rehabilitation.
- Nutrition evaluation and rehabilitation.
- Screening for depression.
- Help with quitting smoking, tobacco use, and alcohol use counseling.

Lymphedema evaluation and rehabilitation.

Age appropriate cancer screenings like lung cancer for smokers and breast cancer.

Age-appropriate vaccinations like HPV vaccines.

Table was generated by author based on review of published literature.

---

met. Planning for ongoing survivorship care should be designed within a year of completion of all treatments.

Recurrent and Second Cancers: Majority of head and neck cancer patients tends to locally recur within 2 to 3 years of follow and should be monitored for these events. Resectable primary cancers should be re-resected with curative intent if feasible, and recurrences in a previously treated neck should undergo surgery as well. Neck disease in an untreated neck should be addressed by formal neck dissection or modification depending on the clinical situation. Non-surgical therapy may also be utilized as clinically appropriate. Survivors of head and neck cancer are susceptible to second cancers and they should always be screened in the clinic for these events.[12] The lung and esophagus are the most common cancers, and they should be enrolled into lung screening trials/protocols. These are more common in patients that continue to smoke and drink during rehabilitation. Patients should be encouraged to quit using tobacco in all forms.[50,51]

SUMMARY

Head and neck cancers are heterogenous cancers with rising incidence of treatable/curative cancers. It is important for clinicians to be aware of managing survivors and the changes induced by therapeutic interventions. As patients live longer, they are more susceptible to delayed effects of multimodal therapy and second cancers. The clinicians should be aware of physiologic and functional changes in vital organs involving daily activities, such as eating, drinking, speech, and communication.

CLINICS CARE POINTS

- Incidence of HPV + oropharynx cancer is rising amongst head and neck cancers.
- Patients with head and neck cancers are best managed by a multi-disciplinary team who address comprehensive needs of patients.
- Patients with head and neck cancer deal with long-term sequelae affecting their quality-of-life and daily activities.
- Second cancers are common in head and neck cancers and primary care providers should be aware of long-term surveillance.

DISCLOSURE

The authors have nothing to disclose.

REFERENCES

1. Chow LQM. Head and neck cancer. N Engl J Med 2020;382(1):60–72, doi: 10.1056.
2. Head Neck Cancers. National comprehensive cancer network guidelines. J Natl Compr Cancer Netw 2022;20(3):224–34. PMID: 35276673.
3. Siegel RL, Miller KD, Wagle NS, et al. Cancer statistics, 2023. CA Cancer J Clin 2023;73:17–48.
4. Chaturvedi AK, Engels EA, Pfeiffer RM, et al. Human papillomavirus and rising oropharyngeal cancer incidence in the United States. J Clin Oncol 2011; 29(32):4294–301.
5. Yu MC, Yuan JM. Nasopharyngeal cancer. In: Schottenfeld D, Fraumeni JF, editors. Cancer epidemiology and prevention. 3rd edition. New York: Oxford University Press; 2006. p. 620–6.
6. Yu MC, Yuan JM. Epidemiology of nasopharyngeal carcinoma. Semin Cancer Biol 2002;12(6):421–9.
7. Adelstein DJ, Ridge JA, Gillison ML, et al. Head and neck squamous cell cancer and the human papillomavirus: summary of a National Cancer Institute State of the Science Meeting, November 9–10, 2008, Washington, D.C. Head Neck 2009;31(11):1393–422.
8. Gandini S, Botteri E, Iodice S, et al. Tobacco smoking and cancer: a meta-analysis. Int J Cancer 2008;122(1):155–64.
9. Hashim D, Genden E, Posner M, et al. Head and neck cancer prevention: from primary prevention to impact of clinicians on reducing burden. Ann Oncol 2019;30(5):744–56.
10. Hashibe M, Brennan P, Chuang SC, et al. Interaction between tobacco and alcohol use and the risk of head and neck cancer: pooled analysis in the International Head and Neck Cancer Epidemiology Consortium. Cancer Epidemiol Biomarkers Prev 2009;18(2):541–50.
11. Goldenberg D, Lee J, Koch WM, et al. Habitual risk factors for head and neck cancer. Otolaryngol Head Neck Surg 2004;131(6):986–93 [PubMed Abstract].
12. Do KA, Johnson MM, Doherty DA, et al. Second primary tumors in patients with upper aerodigestive tract cancers: joint effects of smoking and alcohol (United States). Cancer Causes Control 2003;14(2):131–8.
13. Murshed H. Fundamentals of radiation oncology. Physical, Biological and Clinical Aspects 2019;15:269–316. Third edition. Chapter.

14. Harrison SH. Chapter 14: Head and neck cancer- a multi-disciplinary approach. In: Anatomic lymph nodal levels of the neck. 3rd edition. Philadelphia, PA: Lippincott Williams and Wilkens; 2009. p. 286.
15. Son E, Panwar A, Mosher CH, et al. Cancers of the major salivary gland. J Oncol Pract 2018;14(2):99–108.
16. Horn-Ross PL, Ljung BM, Morrow M. Environmental factors and the risk of salivary gland cancer. Epidemiology 1997;8(4):414–29.
17. Heineman TE, Kuan EC, St John MA. When should surveillance imaging be performed after treatment for head and neck cancer? Laryngoscope 2017;127: 533–4.
18. Mehanna H, Wong WL, McConkey CC, et al. PET-CT surveillance versus neck dissection in advanced head and neck cancer. N Engl J Med 2016;374:1444–54.
19. Ng SP, Pollard C, Berends J, et al. Usefulness of surveillance imaging in patients with head and neck cancer who are treated with definitive radiotherapy. Cancer 2019;125:1823–9.
20. Siegel RL, Miller KD, Fuchs HE, et al. Cancer statistics, 2021. CA A Cancer J Clin 2021;71(1):7–33.
21. Ang KK, Harris J, Wheeler R, et al. Human papillomavirus, and survival of patients with oropharyngeal cancer. N Engl J Med 2010;363(1):24–35.
22. Losser KG, Shah JP, Strong EW. The significance of positive margins in surgically resected epidermoid carcinomas. Head Neck Surg 1978;1:107–11.
23. Haughey BH, Sinha P. Prognostic factors, and survival unique to surgically treated p16+ oropharyngeal cancer. Laryngoscope 2012;122(Suppl 2):S13–33.
24. Fowler J, Campanile Y, Warner A, et al. Surgical margins of the oral cavity: is 5 mm necessary? J Otolaryngol Head Neck Surg 2022;5–38.
25. Hartford AC, Palisca MG, Eichler TJ, et al. American Society for Therapeutic Radiology and Oncology (ASTRO) and American college of Radiology (ACR) practice guidelines for intensity modulated radiation therapy (IMRT). Int J Radiat Oncol Biol Phys 2009;73:9–14.
26. Holmes T, Das R, Lowd. American Society of Radiation Oncology recommendations for documenting intensity – modulated radiation therapy treatments. Int J Radiat Oncol Biol Phys 2009;74:1311–8.
27. Lacas B, Bourhis J, Overgarrd J, et al. Role of radiotherapy fractionation in head neck cancer: an updated meta-analysis. Lacet Oncol 2017;18:1221–37.
28. Stevens CM, Huang SH, Fung S, et al. Retrospective study of palliative radiotherapy in newly diagnosed head neck carcinoma. Int J Radi Oncology bio Physics 2011;81:958–63.
29. Holliday EB, Garden A, Rosenthal D, et al. Proton therapy reduces treatment related toxicities for patients with nasopharyngeal cancer: a case matched control study of intensity modulated proton therapy and intensity modulated photon therapy. Int J Part Thera 2015;2:1–10.
30. Russo AI, Adams Ja, Weyman EA, et al. Long term outcomes after proton beam therapy for sinus and nasal squamous cell caricnomas. Int J rad Onc Bio phys 2016;95:368–76.
31. Bourhis J, Amand C, Pignon J-P. Update of MACH-NC (meta-analysis of chemotherapy in Head neck Cancer) database focused on concomitant chemoradiotherapy. J Clin Oncol, 22 (suppl 14), 2004, Abstract 5505.
32. Pignon JP, Bourhis J, Domenga C. Chemotherapy added to loco regional treatment for Head neck squamous cell carcinoma. Three meta-analyses of updated individual data. MACH-Nc collaborative group. Meta-analysis of chemotherapy on Head neck cancer. Lancet 2000;355:949–55.

33. El -Sayed s, Nelson N. Adjuvant and adjunctive chemotherapy in the management of squamous cell carcinoma of the Head neck region. A meta-analysis of prospective and randomized trials. J Clin Oncol 1996;1196(14):838–47.
34. Ferris RL, Blumenschein Jr G, Fayette G, et al. Nivolumab for recurrent squamous cell carcinoma of the Head and neck. N Eng J Med 2016;375:1856–67.
35. Seiwert TY, Burtness B, Mehra R, et al. Safety and clinical activity of pembroluzimabfor treatment of recurrent or metastatic squamous cell carcinoma of the head and neck : an open label,multicentered Phase 1B trial. Lancet Oncol 2016;17:956–65.
36. Strojan P, Hutcheson KA, Eisbruch A, et al. Treatment of late sequelae after radiotherapy for head and neck cancer. Cancer Treat Rev 2017;59:79–92 [PubMed Abstract].
37. Lochler JL, Bonner JA, Carroll WR, et al. Prophylactic percutaneous endoscipic gastrostomy tube placement in treatment of Head Neck Canecr; a comprehensive review and call for evidence based medicine. J Parental Nutri 2011;35:365–74.
38. Languis JA, Vandijk AM, Doorneart P, et al. More than 10 % weight loss in Head neck cancer patients during Radiotherapy is independently associated with deterioration in quality of life. Nutr Cancer 2013;65:76–83.
39. Talwar B, Donnelly R, Skelly R, et al. Nutritional management in head neck cancer: United Kingdom National multidisciplinary guidelines. J laryngol Oto 2016;130:s32–40.
40. Epstein JB, Barasch A. Oral and Dental health in head and neck cancer patients. Cancer Treat Res 2018;174:43–57.
41. Murdoch-Kinch CA, Zwetchkenbaum S. Dental management of head neck cancer patienttreated with radiation therapy. J Mich Dent Assoc 2011;93:28–37.
42. Jensen Sb, Pedersen AM, Vissink A, et al. A systemic review of salivary gland hypofunction and xerostomia induced by cancer therapies: management strategies' and economic impact. Support Care Cancer 2010;18:1061–79.
43. Bar ADV, Weinstein G, Dutta PR, et al. Gabapentin for treatment of pain syndrome related to radiation induced mucositis in patients with head and neck cancer treated with concurrent chemoradiotherapy. Cancer 2010;116:4206–13.
44. Sio TT, Le-Rademacher JG, Leenstra JL, et al. Effect of Doxepin mouthwash or diphenhydramine-lidocaine-antacid mouthwash vs placebo on radiotherapy related oral mucositis pain: the Aliiance A221304 randomized clinical trial. JAMA 2019;321:1481–90.
45. Mehanna H, Taberna M, Buchwald etal von. Prognostic implications of p16 and HPV discordance in oropharyngeal cancer : a multicenter, multinational individual patient data analysis. Lancet Oncol 2023;24:239–51.
46. Lewis JSJr, beadle B, Bishop JA, et al. Human Papilloma virus testing in head and neck carcinomas. Guidelines from the college of American Pathologists. Arch Pathol lab Med 2018;142–559-597.
47. Gillison ML, D'Souza G, Westra W, et al. Distinct risk factors profiles for human papillomavirus type 16-positive and human papillomavirus type-16 negative head and neck cancers. J Natl Cancer Inst 2008;100(6):407–20.
48. Saraiya M, Unger ER, Thompson TD, et al. US assessment of HPV types in cancers: implications for current and 9-valent HPV vaccines. J Natl Cancer Inst 2015;107(6).
49. Senkomago V, Henley SJ, Thomas CC, et al. Human papillomavirus-attributable cancers - United States, 2012–2016. MMWR. Morbidity and Mortality Weekly Report 2019;68(33):724–8.

50. Argiris A, Brockstein BE, Haraf DJ, et al. Competing causes of death and second primary tumors in patients with locoregionally advanced head and neck cancer treated with chemoradiotherapy. Clin Cancer Res 2004;10(6):1956–62.
51. Chuang SC, Scelo G, Tonita JM, et al. Risk of second primary cancer among patients with head and neck cancers: a pooled analysis of 13 cancer registries. Int J Cancer 2008;123(10):2390–6.

Temporomandibular Junction Disorders

Jennifer Goodfred, DO[a],*, Lauren Simon, MD, MPH[b],
Aysha Azam, DO[c]

KEYWORDS

- Orofacial pain • Temporomandibular junction • Bruxism • Jaw clicking • TC/DMD
- Oral splint • Manual therapy • Non-steroidal anti-inflammatory drugs

KEY POINTS

- Temporomandibular junction disorders (TMD) are a common cause of orofacial pain.
- Diagnosis of TMD is based on history and physical examination findings.
- Validated diagnostic questionnaires can help make the diagnosis of a TMD.
- Non-steroidal anti-inflammatory drugs are an effective first-line treatment for TMDs.
- Manual therapy and home exercises are beneficial for many patients with TMD.

INTRODUCTION

Temporomandibular disorders (TMDs) are common conditions that affect a significant portion of the population. They often present with orofacial or preauricular pain with or without painful jaw motion. Examiners may palpate tenderness in the masticatory muscles or hear or feel a click at the joint with jaw opening and closing. The etiology of this group of conditions can be multifactorial, and the clinical manifestations are variable. A thorough history and careful physical examination are essential for the appropriate diagnosis and treatment of TMDs. The Diagnostic Criteria for TMD (DC/TMD) is a useful evidence-based tool to help assess the condition. Treatments for TMDs range from conservative measures such as analgesics and education to more invasive therapies like surgery. The majority of reports that pain improve over time with non-invasive treatment.

[a] Family Medicine, Department of Family Medicine Baptist Memorial Hospital, 6025 Walnut Grove Road Suite 201, Memphis, TN 38120, USA; [b] Family Medicine, Department of Family Medicine, Loma Linda University Medical Center, 25455 Barton Road, Suite 206A, Loma Linda, CA 92354, USA; [c] Department of Family Medicine, Robert Wood Johnson University Hospital Somerset, 110 Rehill Avenue, Somerville, NJ 08876, USA
* Corresponding author. 6025 Walnut Grove Rd, Suite 201, Memphis, TN 38120.
E-mail address: Jennifer.Goodfred@bmg.md

Prim Care Clin Office Pract 52 (2025) 157–170
https://doi.org/10.1016/j.pop.2024.09.015
0095-4543/25/© 2024 Elsevier Inc. All rights are reserved, including those for text and data mining, AI training, and similar technologies.

HISTORY

Disease of the temporomandibular joint (TMJ) has been recognized and treated by physicians as far back as the 5th century. In the 1930's, otolaryngologist James Costen described the condition as a spectrum of symptoms of the joint, ear, and sinuses. He proposed these symptoms were caused by nerve impingement from mechanical overbite, which contributed to the increasing role of dentists in evaluating the condition. In the 1950's and 1960's, investigators Schwartz and Laskin divided Costen's syndrome into 2 categories: problems of the joint and problems of the muscles. In the 1980's, a group of dentists proposed the umbrella term still in use today: TMDs.[1]

DEFINITIONS

The TMJ is comprised of the mandibular condyle and the glenoid fossa of the temporal bone. A fibrocartilage disk in the middle of the joint is attached to the synovial lined joint capsule.[2] **Fig. 1** demonstrates the relationship of the involved structures. The masticatory muscles that surround the joint are primarily responsible for movement of the joint.[3] **Fig. 2** illustrates the more superficial muscles.

The interplay of joint, muscle, and bone contributes to the different symptoms of the disorder. The National Institute of Dental and Craniofacial Research states that, "TMDs are a group of more than 30 conditions that cause pain and dysfunction in the jaw joint and muscles that control jaw movement."[4]

EPIDEMIOLOGY

The number of people affected by TMDs is difficult to estimate and may vary, based on study methods. In a recent meta-analysis, the global prevalence of TMDs was 34%, was most common in middle aged adults, and more often affected females, as demonstrated in **Fig. 3**.[5]

Another recent analysis found that 4.8% of the United States (US) population reported pain in the region of the TMJ that could relate to a TMD. Prevalence was highest between the ages of 25 and 34 with a slightly higher rate in females. Non-Hispanic and White groups with higher income to poverty ratios were most likely to report jaw or

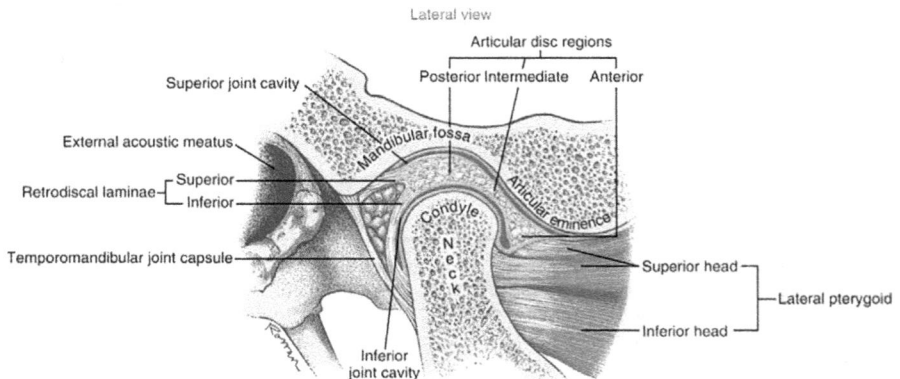

The Temporomandibular Joint (TMJ)- lateral view.

Fig. 1. TMJ Anatomy. Previously published materials unchanged from the source. (Ayşenur Tuncer, Chapter 14 - Kinesiology of the temporomandibular joint, Editor(s): Salih Angin, Ibrahim Engin Şimşek, Comparative Kinesiology of the Human Body, Academic Press, 2020.)

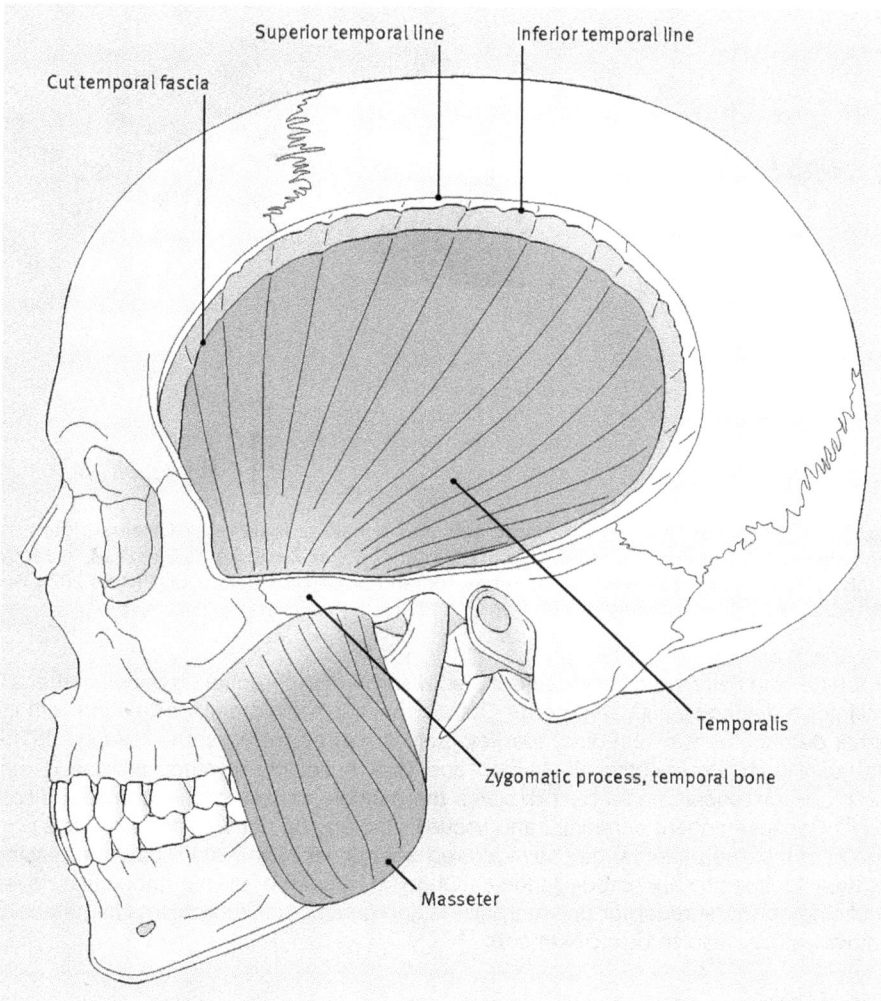

Fig. 2. Muscles. Previously published materials unchanged from the source. (Standring S., Gray's Anatomy: The anatomical basis of clinical practice, 40th edn. Churchill Livingstone, 2008; 538.)

face pain lasting more than 1 day in the 3 months prior to the study.[6] **Table 1** includes socio-demographic data from over 50,000 surveyed US adults from 2017 to 2018. TMDs are the second most common musculoskeletal condition resulting in pain and disability in the US, with an estimated annual cost or 4 billion dollars (about $12 per person in the US.)[7]

ETIOLOGY

The cause and course of development of TMDs have been the subject of much debate, with ideas and research proposed from dentists, allopathic and osteopathic physicians, and physical therapists. TMDs may be divided into intra-articular

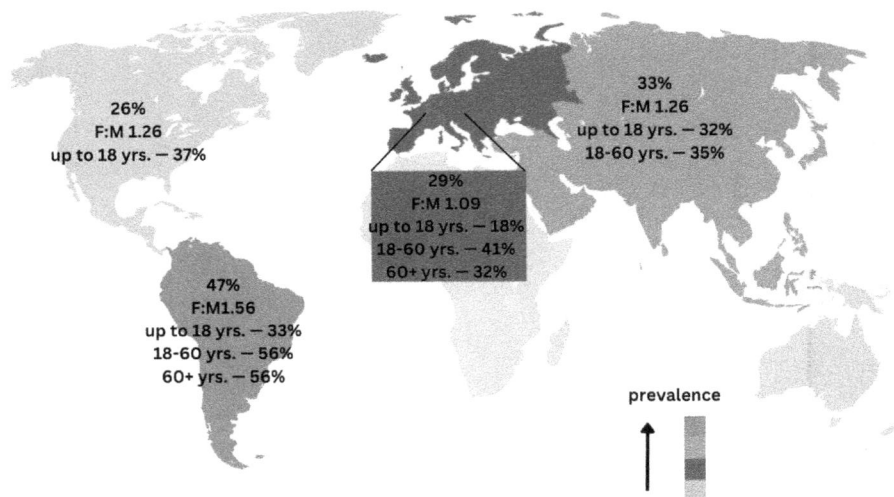

Fig. 3. Prevalence of TMDs by continent, age, and female to male ratio. Original figure using previously published material. (*From* Zielinski G, Pajak-Zielinska B, Ginszt M. A Meta-Analysis of the Global Prevalence of Temporomandibular Disorders. J Clin Med. 2024 Feb 28;13(5):1365. https://doi.org/10.3390/jcm13051365.)

problems and extra-articular muscle-based disorders. Differentiating between these 2 will inform diagnosis and treatment.[8] Osteoarthritic joint changes, correlating with internal derangement of the disc, are key factors addressed by some research.[9] The Orofacial pain: Prospective Evaluation and Risk Assessment study proposed that the biopsychosocial model best explains the multiple causes of this complex disorder.[10] Because patient complaint and tissue pathology do not well correlate, it is proposed that some patients may have altered central nervous system pain processing related to specific inherited genes.[11] Ongoing research at the molecular level, including hormone receptor polymorphisms and genetic polymorphisms in metabolic pathways may lead to new treatments.[12]

DISCUSSION

TMDs may present with symptoms including pain, joint noises, impaired jaw function, and locking. They may overlap with other pain syndromes such as headache and fibromyalgia. This variation contributes to the difficulty diagnosing and treating the condition. Joint noises may lead patients and clinicians to assume a TMD is present, but this assumption may lead to false diagnoses.[13] Because the ear is so close to the TMJ, any joint noise is obvious.[14] Asymptomatic disc displacement (DD) with reduction and without pain is very common and is usually benign, without progression that requires treatment.[15]

TMDs are a leading cause of secondary otalgia in adults. If the history includes clicking with opening the jaw, accompanied by pain, and the physical examination reveals tenderness or crepitus about the joint, a TMD may be present.[16] The most common TMDs include myalgia, myofascial pain, arthralgia, displacements, degenerative joint disease (DJD), subluxation, and headache related to TMD. Intra-articular TMDs involve DD and may occur with or without reduction. They may also include intermittent locking of the joint or limited mouth opening. DJD will have crepitus on

Table 1
Socio-demographic characteristics associated with orofacial pain symptom prevalence in U.S. adults, 2017–2018

Population Group	% of Population	TMD Prevalence* (%, 95% CL)
All adults	100.0	4.8 (4.5, 5.0)
Age (years)		
18–24	11.8	4.2 (3.5, 5.0)
25–34	17.8	4.9 (4.3, 5.4)
35–44	16.4	5.2 (4.6, 5.8)
45–54	16.7	5.4 (4.9, 6.0)
55–64	16.8	5.1 (4.6, 5.7)
65–74	12.1	3.7 (3.3, 4.2)
Sex		
Female	51.7	6.2 (5.9, 6.6)
Male	48.3	3.2 (2.9, 3.5)
Region		
Northeast	17.8	4.4 (3.8, 4.9)
Midwest	21.9	4.9 (4.3, 5.4)
South	36.6	4.5 (4.1, 4.9)
West	23.7	5.4 (4.9, 5.9)
Race		
White	77.7	5.0 (4.8, 5.3)
Black/African American	12.4	3.6 (3.0, 4.2)
Native American	1.2	4.1 (2.8, 5.5)
Asian	6.4	3.0 (2.3, 3.7)
Other/multiple	2.4	7.1 (5.4, 8.8)
Ethnicity		
A: Hispanic	16.2	4.4 (3.8, 5.0)
B: Not Hispanic	83.8	4.8 (4.6, 5.1)
Income: Poverty ratio		
<1.0	10.4	7.3 (6.5, 8.2)
1.0–<2.0	16.1	5.9 (5.3, 6.5)
2.0–<4.0	26.6	4.8 (4.4, 5.2)
≥4.0	40.5	3.7 (3.3, 4.0)
Unknown	6.4	4.5 (3.6, 5.4)

* Jaw or face pain that lasted ≥1 day in the 3 months preceding the NHIS interview. From the authors' analysis of data from n=52,159 participants in the 2017–2018 NHIS surveys.

(National Academies of Sciences, Engineering, and Medicine. 2020. Temporomandibular Disorders: Priorities for Research and Care. https://doi.org/10.17226/25652. Reproduced with permission from the National Academy of Sciences, Courtesy of the National Academies Press, Washington, D.C.)

examination. Subluxation is typically determined by history. Patients with myalgia will present with pain in the jaw, temple, ear, or preauricular region. They will also have pain on palpation of the masseter or temporalis muscles and may also experience pain with mouth opening. Myofascial pain is similar, but spreads beyond the site of palpation and may refer even further beyond the muscle examined. Patients with arthralgia will have pain on palpation of the lateral joint and with mouth opening.

Patients with TMD related headache will have headache pain in the region of the temple that will be worsened with jaw movement.[17]

The majority of TMDs is non-articular and involves muscular dysfunction. Patients may report a history of teeth grinding. Articular diseases such as arthritis and synovitis comprise another portion of disease. Patients with either dysfunction may report dull preauricular pain, joint noises, or restricted jaw motion. Pain that increases with chewing, yawning, or swallowing is considered pathognomonic for TMD. Pain may radiate to the ear or neck and may be made worse by chewing or prolonged opening of the mouth. On examination, the clinician may find joint clicking or locking, tenderness to palpate the muscles or joints, or reduced ability to open the mouth.[18]

Patients with TMD complaints may share other pain conditions such as fibromyalgia, chronic fatigue syndrome, irritable bowel syndrome, chronic back pain, and headaches. TMD and migraine are associated in a bidirectional manner. TMD may cause or exacerbate headaches, which may in turn cause or exacerbate TMDs. The 2 may also be co morbid conditions, and the complex link is the subject of ongoing research.[19] For some patients, particularly those with juvenile arthritis, symptoms may be severe enough to include pain with talking, difficulty eating, and alterations to facial appearance.[14]

TMDs generally involve pain in the face and preauricular areas and may also include limitation to jaw movement. The examiner may find hyperalgesia on palpation of the mastication muscles or the joint and noises with motion.[20] If any red flag signs or symptoms are present, further work up and referral is indicated.[21] Some of those red flags and the differential to consider are included in **Table 2**.

EVALUATION/DIAGNOSIS

TMDs are primarily diagnosed using history and physical examination. The Research Diagnostic Criteria (RDC) for TMDs classified TMD into 3 groups: (i) myogenous/muscular dysfunction/myofascial conditions; (ii) articular disk displacement/derangement; and (iii) articular causes such as arthralgia/arthritis. This broad differential must be considered during the evaluation of TMD to direct appropriate assessment.

The RDC criteria were updated and the recommended evidenced-based DC/TMD was published in 2014. The DC/TMD is used to assess temporomandibular articular and non-articular TMD diagnoses.[17] The DC/TMD has been validated for use in both clinical and research settings to improve diagnostic accuracy for TMD. The DC/TMD diagnostic tool is composed of Axis I and Axis II evaluations, which provide a comprehensive view of the patient's TMD and associated factors. The Axis I evaluations focus on the physical features of TMD diagnoses whereas the Axis II evaluations focus on the psychosocial and pain-related disability assessments of temporomandibular diagnoses.

Axis I assesses for features such as joint noise during TMJ use, grinding, pain, and functional limitations such as reduced mandibular range of motion or reduced jaw opening (less than 35 mm), jaw locking or popping, pain in muscles of mastication, headache, and problems chewing or occlusal problems.[22] (Yadav) Axis II evaluates psychosocial aspects of TMD, such as anxiety, depression, pain-related disability, and quality of life.[23] Axis II assessment, which detects pain-related psychosocial functioning with TMD, includes 5 self-report screening tests: Patient health quesionaire-4, Graded chronic pain scale, a pain drawing of head jaw and body, the Jaw Functional Limitation Scale and Oral Behaviors Checklist.

The DC/TMD outlines diagnostic criteria for the 12 common TMDs including the pain-related disorders of myalgia and types of myalgia differentiated with palpation:

Table 2
Red flags that require special attention in the assessment of TMD/headache patients

Red Flag	Differential diagnoses to consider
History of malignancy	Malignancy recurrence
Presence of lymphadenopathy or neck masses	Neoplastic, infective, or autoimmune cause
Sensory or motor function changes (specifically focusing on cranial nerves V, VII, and VIII)	Intracranial causes, or malignancy affecting the nerve's peripheral branches
Recurrent epistaxis, purulent nasal drainage, or anosmia	Nasopharyngeal carcinoma or chronic sinusitis
Trismus	Oral malignancy
Unexplained fever, fatigue, weight loss	Malignant tumors, immunosuppression, and infective causes
Facial asymmetry or masses	Neoplastic, infective, or inflammatory causes
Occlusal changes	Growth disturbance of condyle, neoplasia, rheumatoid arthritis, and traumatic causes
Ipsilateral objective change in hearing	Acoustic neuroma, or other ear disease
Neurologic symptoms (confusion, aphasia, dysarthria)	Artery dissection, intracranial hemorrhage
History of recent head and neck trauma	Arterial dissection, intracranial hemorrhage
Sudden onset headache	Subarachnoid hemorrhage
Postural or positional aggravation	Increased/Decreased intracranial pressure (idiopathic intracranial hypertension, meningitis)
Onset >50 years of age + jaw claudication	Temporal arteritis
Persisting or worsening symptoms despite treatment	Misdiagnosis or more complex case

(From Kapos FP, Exposto FG, Oyarzo JF, Durham J. Temporomandibular disorders: a review of current concepts in aetiology, diagnosis and management. Oral Surg. 2020;13(4):321-334. doi:10.1111/ors.12473.)

local myalgia, myofascial pain and myofascial pain with referral; arthralgia, Intra-articular TMD of 4 DD disorders, DJD, joint subluxation and headache associated with TMD. **Box 1** lists common descriptions of the myalgia pain disorder of TMD. Although most of the TMD disorders are diagnosed by history and physical examination, MRI imaging of the TMJs is required to confirm diagnosis of TMJ DD (except for DD without reduction with limited opening/"closed-lock" can be diagnosed without imaging) and computed tomography (CT) is needed to confirm TMJ DJD.[17] Although MRI imaging is considered the standard to assess TMD, it is expensive and not always available. TMD may be asymptomatic early in the disease even while joint damage can occur. The DC/TMD criteria outline imaging findings, which are often present late in TMD such as condylar damage, osteophytes, surface erosions, and sclerosis. Ultrasound can also be used to diagnose internal derangement of the TMJ but the sensitivity and specificity is currently not superior to MRI for these evaluations. One major advantage of using ultrasound is it captures dynamic views of the TMJ during function.[24] Although ultrasound is useful for evaluating DD in TMD, advanced imaging with CT/Cone Beam CT are needed as a reference standard to determine validity for use of ultrasound to assess condylar changes.[25] Currently MRI is used for these TMD assessments.

Box 1
Description of myalgia and myalgia subtypes of pain related temporomandibular disorders

Myalgia
- Pain of muscle origin that is affected by jaw movement, function or parafunction and replication of this pain occurs with provocation pain with testing of the masticatory muscles. (Schiffman)
- Pain occurs in ear, front of ear, jaw, or temple and is modified with jaw movement or function/parafunction for myalgia and the subtypes of myalgia: local myalgia; myofascial pain and myofascial pain with referral:

Local myalgia
- Pain of muscle origin that is affected by jaw movement, function or parafunction and replication of this pain occurs with provocation pain with testing of the masticatory muscles.
- Localization of pain only at site of palpation when using the myofascial examination protocol (Schiffman, Orbach)

Myofascial pain
- Pain of muscle origin that is affected by jaw movement, function or parafunction and replication of this pain occurs with provocation pain with testing of the masticatory muscles. Pain spreading beyond site of palpation but within boundary of the muscle when using the myofascial examination protocol (Schiffman, Orbach)

Myofascial pain with referral
- Pain of muscle origin that is affected by jaw movement, function or parafunction and replication of this pain occurs with provocation pain with testing of the masticatory muscles. Pain spreading beyond site of palpation but within boundary of the muscle when using the myofascial examination protocol (Schiffman, Orbach) Spreading pain may be present.

Original Box using previously published data: *Data from* Ohrbach R, Gonzalez YM, List T, Michelotti A, Schiffman EL. [7/28/2013]; *Diagnostic Criteria for Temporomandibular Disorders (DC/TMD) Clinical Examination Protocol.* http://www.rdc-tmdinternational.org/Portals/18/protocol_DC-TMD/DC-TMDProtocol-2013_06_02.pdf.

Physical assessment for TMD should include a head and neck evaluation and evaluation of the jaw/TMJ joint and associated structures palpating for crepitus and tenderness and listening for joint noise and assessment for mouth opening. The examiner should observe the patient for postural deficits and general size, shape, and symmetry of the mandible; observe active range of motion on mouth opening and jaw deviation, and protrusion.[23,26] If applicable, passive accessory motion can be checked with the gloved hand of the examiner.[26] The clinical examination to diagnose arthralgia includes testing for pain provocation with any jaw movements and palpation of the TMJ, anterior to the tragus bilaterally. In those with known or suspected inflammatory arthritis such as, juvenile idiopathic arthritis, rheumatoid arthritis, psoriatic arthritis, Ankylosing Spondylitis or Sjogren's, which may include TMD arthropathy, a broader physical assessment is advised.[24,27]

For myalgia diagnosis, the history includes pain in the jaw, temple ear or in front of the ear, and pain modified with jaw movement, function, or parafunction plus confirmation of pain location. The physical examination testing includes pain on palpation of the temporalis and masseter muscles, best performed with patient in clenched teeth position[3] along with pain on jaw palpation or opening.[17] The masseters are palpated with fingers pressing over the angle of the mandible. The temporalis muscles are palpated along the temple with the jaw relaxed and clenched.[28] Both diagnoses of DD with reduction and DJD require positive joint crepitus or popping during the clinical examination to confirm the diagnoses.[17] Clicking occurs when the TMJ articular disc moves anterior to the condylar head and popping sound may occur when the disk moves back into position.[3]

In addition to inflammatory arthritis,[29–31] the history and clinical examination for TMD should include consideration for other disorders, which can mimic TMD pain such as dental caries, trigeminal neuralgia sinusitis, herpes zoster, giant cell arteritis, cancer, or autoimmune disease such as systemic lupus erythematosus.[9]

TREATMENT

The "Best Practices in Oral Surgery" recommendation from Choosing Wisely emphasizes the importance of avoiding invasive therapies for TMD early in the treatment course. They recommend avoiding irreversible surgical procedures such as braces, occlusal equilibration, and restorations, as first-line treatments.[32] To address the multifaceted nature of TMDs, the best treatment supports a combination of pharmacologic and non-pharmacologic therapies, along with patient education and self-care strategies.

NON-PHARMACOLOGIC THERAPY

Empowering patients through education and self-care is a key component of the initial therapy for TMDs. Self-management strategies including optimal head posture, sleep hygiene, avoidance of triggers (like nail biting, chewing gum, clenching, and grinding), heat or ice, a soft food diet, and home exercises, can significantly contribute to the management of TMD.[33] Because of the potential for benefit with little harm, educating patients on these self-care measures is recommended despite low-quality evidence.[32]

For patients with comorbid depression, anxiety, or stress disorders, biobehavioral management can be used as an adjunctive therapy. Modalities such as biofeedback and cognitive behavioral therapy (CBT) resulted in short-term improvement and reduced medication usage. A meta-analysis including 15 trials of patients with TMD, CBT—alone or with biofeedback—resulted in long-term improvement in activity. However, the meta-analysis was limited by the small number of high-quality trials.[32]

Physical therapy plays a significant role in the management of TMJ disorders, particularly for patients with a musculoskeletal component like neck or shoulder symptoms. Manual therapy, where therapists use their hands to decrease pain and joint dysfunction through direct pressure on the muscles and joints, is standard. Therapy may include TMJ mobilization and stability, massage, and patient posture evaluation. Physical therapy may improve pain and function, but the evidence is unclear.[32] The lack of high-quality evidence is due to the methodologic issues limiting comparison between the studies. In patients with bruxism, an occlusal splint fitted by a dentist can be used with other therapies, especially physical therapy.[33] However, the evidence supporting occlusal splints is mixed; some systematic reviews show a benefit, while others show no improvement.

PHARMACOLOGIC THERAPY

Although non-steroidal anti-inflammatory drugs (NSAIDs) and muscle relaxers are used for a wide variety of acute and chronic pain disorders, there is a lack of high-quality evidence supporting the efficacy in treating chronic TMD. A systematic review of 4 randomized controlled trials showed that NSAIDs decreased pain.[32] However, due to the variability of the study protocols, the review concluded with only moderate certainty that this improvement was clinically meaningful. The overall recommendation is to use NSAIDs at the lowest effective dose for the shortest duration. Cardiovascular and gastrointestinal risk factors should be assessed before prescribing NSAIDs. Naproxen, 500 mg twice daily for 10 to 14 days, decreased pain significantly and increased the range of motion in patients compared to the placebo.[32] For patients unable to take oral NSAIDs, topical diclofenac—which should also be limited to a 14-day course—massaged over the joint and muscle can be helpful in pain reduction. Acetaminophen can also be used—650 mg every 6 hours as needed—to relieve pain.[32] However, as acetaminophen does not have anti-inflammatory properties, it may be less effective.

Skeletal muscle relaxants can be used for patients with palpable tenderness of the mastication muscles. Skeletal muscle relaxers should be taken on a schedule instead of on an as-needed basis. Cyclobenzaprine, 10 mg nightly for 3 weeks, decreased pain compared to the placebo based on 1 network meta-analysis.[32] Cyclobenzaprine is recommended to be taken at night due to its sedating quality. A lower dose should be started and gradually increased for patients more sensitive to the sedating quality. Cyclobenzaprine is not recommended for long-term use. An alternative for daytime use would be metaxalone, 400 mg every 8 hours.[32]

For patients with persistent pain, even after 2 weeks of NSAID therapy or 3 w of skeletal muscle relaxants, the next line of treatment is tricyclic antidepressants (TCAs).[34] Amitriptyline, 25 mg nightly for 2 weeks, reduced pain by 35% compared to 14% with the placebo.[32] Nortriptyline can be used if the patient experiences anticholinergic side effects with amitriptyline. Nortriptyline, starting at 10 mg nightly, can be titrated up to 25 mg nightly. A dose over 25 mg is not recommended due to side effects.[34] An adequate treatment trial can take up to 6 to 12 weeks. The dosage is reduced for the patients who respond adequately, and the patient is continued on the lowest effective dosage for up to 4 mo. TCAs should be avoided in patients with cardiac conduction abnormalities. Diazepam did show effectiveness in one study. However, it should be avoided due to the risk of addiction and modest improvement.[32] Opioids are not recommended due to the high risk of dependence and the availability of other treatment options.

OSTEOPATHIC MANUAL THERAPY

There are several techniques to treat TMDs with osteopathic manipulative medicine. These include muscle energy technique (MET), myofascial release (MFR), and balanced ligamentous tension (BLT). MET is a technique that engages the restrictive barriers of the muscle. The patient would apply muscle effort in a specific direction, meeting a counterforce applied by the practitioner.[35] MET can lengthen muscles and mobilize the restricted joint.[35] MFR is a passive technique in which the physician palpates the tight or restricted fascia and stretches the soft tissue.[35] This will allow the tissue and joint to become looser. BLT is an active and passive technique that exaggerates the dysfunction to help guide muscle movement. Osteopathic manual therapy (OMT) effectively moves the dysfunctional joint complex through the restrictive barrier. A study comparing OMT versus conventional conservative therapy demonstrated that the patients who received OMT required significantly less medicatio.[36]

Contraindications of MET include low vitality, jaw fractures, unstable joints, and recent surgery.[35] Contraindications for MFR include healing fractures, advanced diabetes, severe osteoporosis, rheumatoid arthritis, malignancy, and aneurysm.[35] Contraindications of BLT include acute jaw fractures, temporal bone malignancy, and a history of osteomyelitis.[35]

INJECTIONS

Patients with temporomandibular joint osteoarthritis may benefit from an intra-articular injection. Glucocorticoid injections can provide symptomatic pain relief for up to

6 months. Corticosteroid injections are limited to 2 or 3 times, separated by 4 to 6 weeks. Intra-articular corticosteroid injections are not routinely recommended due to the potential for destruction of the articular cartilage. However, these injections are reserved for some patients with severe arthritic changes. Intra-articular injections with hyaluronic acid or platelet-rich plasma can be considered; however, a consistent long-term benefit has not been seen.[37] Botulinum toxin can be injected into the masseter and temporalis muscles for patients with predominantly musculoskeletal pain. This injection can be combined with long-acting anesthesia trigger point injections into the temporalis tendon. A systematic review found that botulinum toxin injections decreased myalgias but not arthralgias.[32]

ALTERNATIVE THERAPY

Dry and wet needling within the muscles decreased pain in one systematic review. However, high-quality clinical trials using an active control group receiving sham therapy are needed. Acupuncture relieved myofascial pain in one retrospective cohort study; however, there was no comparison group. Low-level laser therapy has shown positive effects in pain relief in 18 out of 30 studies in one systematic review. However, due to the variability in the study protocols, additional trials are needed before laser therapy can be recommended. In a meta-analysis, glucosamine was shown to be as effective as ibuprofen at 12 weeks for pain control. However, only 1 of the 3 studies was of high quality.[32]

PROGNOSIS

TMD is self-limiting in the general population, and most patients will respond well to treatment. Almost 90% of patients with TMD will respond to noninvasive treatments.[32]

SUMMARY

TMDs are prevalent in primary and specialty care in the US and around the world. Painful conditions of the temporomandibular joint have been evaluated and treated by generations of doctors, dentists, and therapists. The terminology has changed, and the etiology and pathogenesis have been studied and debated. Epidemiologic data have been collected and published. Diagnostic tools have been developed and revised, and treatments have expanded beyond medication or surgery to include complementary and alternative therapies. To provide quality care for patients suffering with a TMD, a careful history and physical examination performed by an informed clinician are essential for accurate diagnosis of this multifaceted condition. Recognition of the biopsychosocial components that are associated with TMD dysfunction is equally important. Many patients with TMD will improve with time and conservative measures. For the small percentage of patients with a more complicated presentation or course, specialty testing and treatment are available, and research is ongoing.

CLINICS CARE POINTS

- TMDs involve pain around the TMJ and muscles of mastication.
- Some patients with TMD will have associated orofacial pain, otalgia, or headache.
- Clicking or popping of the joint upon mouth opening with or without pain is a common complaint.
- Most TMDs are non-articular.

- The prevalence of TMD is greatest in middle aged females.
- Utilization of the RD/TMD facilitates accurate diagnosis of TMDs.
- Conservative therapy with analgesics is the best initial treatment for most TMDs.
- Best practice is to avoid invasive therapy as initial treatment for TMDs.

DISCLOSURES

The authors have nothing to disclose.

REFERENCES

1. Laskin DM. Temporomandibular disorders: a term whose time has passed. J Oral Maxillofac Surg 2020;78(4):496–7.
2. Stocum DL, Roberts WE. Part I: development and physiology of the temporomandibular joint. Curr Osteoporos Rep 2018;16(4):360–8.
3. Gauer R, Semidy M. Diagnosis and treatment of temporomandibular disorders. Am Fam Physician 2015;91(6):378–86.
4. NIH. TMD (Temporomandibular Disorders). www.nidcr.nih.gov. Published March 2023. Available at: https://www.nidcr.nih.gov/health-info/tmd (Accessed 8 April 2024).
5. Zielinski G, Pajak-Zielinska B, Ginszt M. A meta-analysis of the global prevalence of temporomandibular disorders. J Clin Med 2024;13(5):1365.
6. Bond EC, Mackey S, English R, et al. In: Temporomandibular disorders. Washington, DC: National Academies Press; 2020.
7. Facial pain. Available at: www.nidcr.nih.gov. https://www.nidcr.nih.gov/research/data-statistics/facial-pain (Accessed 8 April 2024).
8. Mercuri LG. Temporomandibular joint facts and foibles. J Clin Med 2023;12(9):3246.
9. Murphy MK, MacBarb RF, Wong ME, et al. Temporomandibular disorders: a review of etiology, clinical management, and tissue engineering strategies. Int J Oral Maxillofac Implants 2013;28(6):e393–414.
10. Slade GD, Fillingim RB, Sanders AE, et al. Summary of findings from the OPPERA prospective cohort study of incidence of first-onset temporomandibular disorder: implications and future directions. J Pain 2013;14(12):T116–24.
11. Cairns BE. Pathophysiology of TMD pain - basic mechanisms and their implications for pharmacotherapy. J Oral Rehabil 2010;37(6):391–410.
12. Durham J, Newton-John TRO, Zakrzewska JM. Temporomandibular disorders. BMJ 2015;350(mar12 9):h1154.
13. Moxley B, Stevens W, Sneed J, et al. Novel diagnostic and therapeutic approaches to temporomandibular dysfunction: a narrative review. Life 2023;13(9):1808.
14. Stoll ML, Kau CH, Waite PD, et al. Temporomandibular joint arthritis in juvenile idiopathic arthritis, now what? Pediatr Rheumatol Online J 2018;16(1):32.
15. Poluha RL, Canales GT, Costa YM, et al. Temporomandibular joint disc displacement with reduction: a review of mechanisms and clinical presentation [published correction appears in J Appl Oral Sci. 2019 Apr 01;27:e2019er001]. J Appl Oral Sci 2019;27:e20180433.
16. Earwood JS, Rogers TS, Rathjen NA. Ear pain: diagnosing common and uncommon causes. Am Fam Physician 2018;97(1):20–7.

17. Schiffman E, Ohrbach R, Truelove E, et al, International RDC/TMD Consortium Network, International association for Dental Research; Orofacial Pain Special Interest Group, International Association for the Study of Pain. Diagnostic criteria for temporomandibular disorders (DC/TMD) for clinical and research applications: recommendations of the International RDC/TMD consortium network* and orofacial pain special interest group. J Oral Facial Pain Headache 2014;28(1):6–27. Winter.

18. Ghazal F, Ahmad M, Elrawy H, et al. Zeroing in on the cause of your patient's facial pain. J Fam Pract 2015;64(9):524–531B.

19. Yakkaphan Pankaew, Elias LA, Priya Thimma Ravindranath, et al. Is painful temporomandibular disorder a real headache for many patients? Br Dent J 2024;236(6):475–82.

20. Ohrbach R, Dworkin SF. The evolution of TMD diagnosis. J Dent Res 2016;95(10):1093–101.

21. Kapos FP, Exposto FG, Oyarzo JF, et al. Temporomandibular disorders: a review of current concepts in aetiology, diagnosis and management. Oral Surg 2020;13(4):321–34.

22. Yadav S, Yang Y, Dutra EH, et al. Temporomandibular joint disorders in older adults. J Am Geriatr Soc 2018;66(6):1213–7. Epub 2018 May 2. PMID: 29719041; PMCID: PMC6699643.

23. Minervini G, Franco R, Marrapodi MM, et al. Correlation between temporomandibular disorders (TMD) and posture evaluated trough the diagnostic criteria for temporomandibular disorders (DC/TMD): a systematic review with meta-analysis. J Clin Med 2023;12(7):2652. PMID: 37048735; PMCID: PMC10095000.

24. Maranini B, Giovanni C, Stefano M, et al. The role of ultrasound in temporomandibular joint disorders: an update and future perspectives. Front Med 2022. https://doi.org/10.3389/fmed.2022.926573.

25. Almeida F, Pacheco-Pereira C, Flores-Mir C, et al. Diagnostic ultrasound assessment of temporomandibular joints: a systematic review and meta-analysis. Dentomaxillofacial Radiol 2019;48(2):20180144.

26. Shaffer SM, Brismée JM, Sizer PS, et al. Temporomandibular disorders. Part 1: anatomy and examination/diagnosis. J Man Manip Ther 2014;22(1):2–12. PMID: 24976743; PMCID: PMC4062347.

27. Rongo R, Ekberg E, Nilsson IM, et al. Diagnostic criteria for temporomandibular disorders (DC/TMD) for children and adolescents: an international Delphi study-Part 1-Development of Axis I. J Oral Rehabil 2021;48(7):836–45. Epub 2021 May 19. PMID: 33817818; PMCID: PMC8252391.

28. Liu F, Steinkeler A. Epidemiology, diagnosis, and treatment of temporomandibular disorders. Dent Clin North Am 2013;57(3):465–79. PMID: 23809304.

29. Peck CC, Goulet JP, Lobbezoo F, et al. Expanding the taxonomy of the diagnostic criteria for temporomandibular disorders. J Oral Rehabil 2014;41(1):2–23. PMID: 24443898; PMCID: PMC4520529.

30. Tuncer A. Kinesiology of the temporomandibular joint. Cambridge, MA: Elsevier eBooks; 2020.

31. Slade G, Durham J. Prevalence, impact, and costs of treatment for temporomandibular disorders. Paper commissioned by the committee on temporomandibular disorders (TMDs): from research discoveries to clinical treatment. In temporomandibular disorders: priorities for research and care (see appendix C). Washington, DC: the national academies press. National academies of sciences, engineering, and medicine. 2020. Temporomandibular disorders: priorities for

research and care. Washington, DC: The National Academies Press; 2020. https://doi.org/10.17226/25652.

32. Matheson EM, Fermo JD, Blackwelder RS. Temporomandibular disorders: rapid evidence review. Am Fam Physician 2023;107(1):52–8.

33. Eliassen M, Hjortsjö C, Olsen-Bergem H, et al. Self-exercise programmes and occlusal splints in the treatment of TMD-related myalgia—evidence-based medicine? J Oral Rehabil 2019;(11):1088–94.

34. Rizzatti-Barbosa CM, Nogueira MTP, de Andrade ED, et al. Clinical evaluation of amitriptyline for the control of chronic pain caused by temporomandibular joint disorders. CRANIO® 2003;(3):221–5.

35. Nahian A, Unal M, Matthew J, Osteopathic manipulative treatment: facial muscle energy, direct MFR, and BLT procedure – for TMJ dysfunction - StatPearls - NCBI Bookshelf, 2023, National Center for Biotechnology Information; Treasure Island, FL. Available at: https://www.ncbi.nlm.nih.gov/books/NBK564310/ (Accessed 7 May 2024).

36. Cuccia AM, Caradonna C, Annunziata V, et al. Osteopathic manual therapy versus conventional conservative therapy in the treatment of temporomandibular disorders: a randomized controlled trial. J Bodyw Mov Ther 2010;(2):179–84.

37. Al-Moraissi EA, Wolford LM, Ellis E, et al. The hierarchy of different treatments for arthrogenous temporomandibular disorders: a network meta-analysis of randomized clinical trials. J Cranio-Maxillofacial Surg 2020;(1):9–23.

Dysphagia

Gretchen M. Irwin, MD, MBA*, Jordan Leatherman, MD

KEYWORDS

- Dysphagia • Impaired swallow • Oropharyngeal dysfunction
- Esophageal dysfunction

KEY POINTS

- Dysphagia is a symptom of an underlying pathology, not a disease unto itself.
- Many patients will not report dysphagia; yet, symptoms have significant quality of life impacts.
- Determining if dysphagia is resulting from oropharyngeal or esophageal dysfunction will guide diagnostic workup.
- Esophagogastroduodenoscopy is the diagnostic intervention of choice for esophageal dysphagia.

BACKGROUND

Dysphagia, defined as impairment of the swallowing mechanism, that may affect 1 in 6 adults and can be associated with significant morbidity and mortality.[1,2] Dysphagia affects quality of life as patients may adapt their eating with prolonged eating times or excessive liquid intake.[2,3] Despite symptom severity or need for intervention only half of individuals experiencing symptoms seek medical care.[2] Without proper intervention, patients may avoid eating or develop feelings of isolation and embarrassment.[4]

Each year approximately 1 million new cases of dysphagia are diagnosed in the United States with an estimated annual cost of $4 to $7 million dollars according to a study.[5,6] Although dysphagia can occur at any age, up to 13% of patients older than 65 years may experience dysphagia.[7]

Swallowing requires the coordination of complex brain signals, 6 cranial nerves and 50 pairs of striated cranial muscles in the space of a few seconds.[8,9] First, food is chewed and a bolus is formed by skeletal muscle under voluntary control during the oral phase.[9] Next, voluntary and involuntary processes are involved to move the bolus into the pharynx and close the airway during the pharyngeal phase.[9,10] Finally, food passes through the esophagus via slow peristaltic contractions that may take up to

Department of Family and Community Medicine, University of Kansas School of Medicine-Wichita, 1010 North Kansas, Wichita, KS 67214, USA
* Corresponding author.
E-mail address: Girwin2@kumc.edu

Prim Care Clin Office Pract 52 (2025) 171–179
https://doi.org/10.1016/j.pop.2024.09.016
0095-4543/25/© 2024 Elsevier Inc. All rights reserved, including those for text and data mining, AI training, and similar technologies.

10 seconds to move the bolus toward the stomach.[8–10] Because of the complexity of this process, multiple pathologic processes may cause dysphagia.

CLINICAL PRESENTATION

Physicians should remember that dysphagia is a symptom, not a disease unto itself; therefore, investigation to determine and potentially treat the underlying cause is critical. A variety of etiologies may lead to dysphagia, and a good clinical history is the first step in pursuing proper treatment.

Dysphagia may be divided into oropharyngeal and esophageal forms. Oropharyngeal dysphagia is commonly caused by neurologic conditions, such as Parkinson's disease, dementia, cerebrovascular ischemia, or malignancy and may be a presenting sign of amyotrophic lateral sclerosis or myasthenia gravis.[9,11–13] Esophageal dysphagia may be caused by gastroesophageal reflux disease, eosinophilic esophagitis, esophageal strictures, webs or ring, achalasia, medications, infections, or rheumatologic conditions such as scleroderma.[4,9]

Differentiating oropharyngeal and esophageal dysphagia may be aided by careful analysis of patient symptoms. Difficulty chewing, trouble initiating a swallow, coughing, choking, a wet sounding voice following a swallow, or nasopharyngeal regurgitation suggest oropharyngeal causes.[4,9] Esophageal causes are suggested when patients describe a feeling of food getting stuck once swallowing has occurred.[9] This should be differentiated from globus pharyngeus which is the sensation of something caught in the throat that improves with swallowing.[14] Patients with esophageal dysphagia may accurately localize an obstruction to the mid or lower chest; however, patients may also report feeling food trapped in the throat when, in reality, the lesion is much lower and the patient is misled by overlapping sensory innervation.[15,16] Additional clues to esophageal dysfunction can include regurgitation of undigested food which suggests achalasia or a Zenker diverticulum while painful swallowing suggests infection such as candidiasis.[4] Similarly, a history of asthma or food allergies may suggest eosinophilic esophagitis as a cause of symptoms.[4]

One key history element to elicit is if dysphagia occurs with swallowing solids, liquids, or both. Dysphagia resulting from mechanical obstructions that worsen over time, such as strictures or malignancy, tends to present with difficulty swallowing solid foods that progresses to difficulty with solids and liquids.[9] Patients who experience difficulty with both solids and liquids at the onset of symptoms tend to have esophageal motility issues such as achalasia.[4,9] Further, dysphagia resulting from a neurologic or oropharyngeal cause tends to present with difficulty swallowing liquids first as evidenced by coughing or choking when drinking.[4,8]

The onset and duration of dysphagia can give clues to the etiology as well. Patients presenting with acute symptoms may have esophagitis, infection, or foreign body impaction.[4]

Rapidly progressing dysphagia over weeks to months may be indicative of malignancy whereas peptic stricture should be considered with lower progression in the setting of reflux.[1,17] Intermittent dysphagia over the course of years is most likely associated with a benign etiology such as esophageal web or eosinophilic esophagitis.[18]

Medication review is critical to fully evaluate patients presenting with dysphagia. Patients utilizing proton pump inhibitors or histamine-2 blockers may have underlying gastroesophageal reflux disease causing dysphagia.[4] Too, non-steroidal anti-inflammatory medications or bisphosphonates can contribute to pill-induced esophagitis while anti-cholinergic or anti-muscarinic medications may worsen xerostomia and difficulty initiating swallow.[1,4,9] Tricyclic anti-depressants may worsen reflux symptoms and increase dysphagia symptoms, though some evidence suggests that amitriptyline (25 mg) or imipramine (50 mg) may improve dyspepsia symptoms.[19] Sedatives that reduce attention or cause drowsiness as well as steroids which may weaken tongue strength can also lead to an impaired swallow.[9]

Opioids are an important medication to consider when evaluating dysphagia as increasing potency and 24-hour morphine equivalent doses are frequently associated with esophageal dysfunction and dysphagia.[20] This opioid-induced esophageal dysmotility may improve with cessation of opioid medications or dose reductions, though evidence is lacking to guide optimal therapy.[20]

In addition to history, a thorough physical examination may yield clues to determine the cause of dysphagia. Neurologic examination may reveal subtle findings suggesting a neurologic syndrome of which dysphagia is a feature. Examination of cranial nerve function, soft palate elevation, tongue mobility, jaw movement, and voice changes with swallow can provide important clues to the cause of dysphagia.[8,21] A simple observation of ill-fitting dentures or dry mouth may elucidate an easily remedied cause of difficulty swallowing.[4] However, in the ambulatory environment, physicians may be limited in the ability to observe a patient swallowing liquids and solids of various textures or to directly visualize the larynx and esophagus. Thus, while an important source of information to direct the workup, physical examination alone will likely not diagnose all underlying causes of dysphagia.[1]

CLINICAL WORKUP

When oropharyngeal dysphagia is suspected based upon history and physical examination, a speech and language pathologist may be an important health care team member to involve in the care of the patient.[1] Patients often undergo bedside swallow evaluations which include a thorough history and physical examination as well as administration of various sizes, textures, and types of food.[9] Such bedside swallow examinations can provide important information to help elucidate a diagnosis, though insufficient evidence exists to utilize bedside evaluations alone to determine optimal treatment.[22,23] Direct visualization of the vocal cords can also assist to diagnose oropharyngeal dysphagia, particularly if related to structural masses or lesions.[24]

Esophagogastroduodenoscopy (EGD) may be the most effective tool for evaluating suspected esophageal swallowing disorders, especially in patients older than 40 years of age.[25] It provides the best direct visualization of tissues, and it allows for direct mucosal biopsies. Biopsies should be taken to evaluate for malignant pathology and eosinophilic esophagitis.[26] Endoscopy also allows for immediate, therapeutic intervention with dilation if indicated.[1]

Videofluoroscopic swallowing studies may be beneficial if both oropharyngeal and esophageal causes are suspected.[9] Such studies allow for evaluation of both structure and function of relevant anatomic structures and are the studies of choice when evaluation of the swallowing mechanism and peristalsis is sought.[27] Modified barium swallow studies are preferred over endoscopy to detect subtle narrowing or webs.[4] In addition to the videofluoroscopic studies, fiberoptic endoscopic evaluation of swallowing study may be recommend if there is concern for silent aspiration, as it is most useful to evaluate management of secretions.[17]

DISCUSSION

Dysphagia can result in significant morbidity and mortality related to aspiration pneumonia and malnutrition, particularly in elderly patients and those presenting with neurologic disease[24,28] Management is directed at identifying the underlying cause and providing treatment of that cause when possible. Behavioral, pharmacologic, and surgical interventions may be helpful depending on the underlying cause of the dysphagia symptoms.[29–31] Behavioral interventions may include recommendations about posture when eating, food size, food texture, sequence of solid and liquids when eating, or exercises designed to improve voluntarily controlled muscles of swallowing. These all have been shown to have varying degrees of improvement of dysphagia and patient adherence depending on the underlying condition, patient population, and intervention recommended.[32] Use of food thickeners, for example, has been shown to have decreasing patient adherence over time with inconsistent definitions of food consistency across geographic locations and institutions limiting generalizability of research findings.[33,34]

Gastroesophageal Reflux Disease/Acid Reflux

Gastroesophageal reflux disease (GERD) is the most common etiology of swallowing disorders and up to 32% of patients with GERD have frequent dysphagia.[11,35] Young patients who do not have alarming symptoms, such as weight loss or pain with dysphagia, may be presumptively treated for GERD with 4 weeks of proton pump inhibitor therapy to see if dysphagia resolves before proceeding with EGD.[36,37] However, dysphagia should be considered an alarming symptom if it develops in older patients with GERD and warrants immediate endoscopy.[38] Long-term erosive esophagitis may lead to the formation of peptic strictures, which form in the healing process.[35] Too severe inflammation as a result of GERD can lead to Barrett's esophagitis which may also present with dysphagia in the first stages of esophageal cancer.[38]

Eosinophilic Esophagitis

Eosinophilic esophagitis is becoming an increasing cause of dysphagia and is currently the leading cause of emergent food impaction in the United States.[39] Dysphagia occurs as the result of both narrowing and dysmotility in the esophagus. Physicians should ensure that biopsies are taken from the proximal and distal esophagus during EGD to best assess for this.[35] Typically treatment of this condition requires diets which eliminate allergens and/or topical steroids for maximal benefit.[40,41]

Neurologic Disorders

Neurologic diseases such as stroke, neurodegenerative diseases, dementia, myopathies, peripheral neuropathies, and motor neuron disease may lead to oropharyngeal dysphagia. Globally, up to 800,000 individuals develop neurogenic dysphagia each year, including up to 65% of patients with acute cerebrovascular ischemia, 50% of patients with Parkinson's disease, and 31% of patients with multiple sclerosis.[8,42] Early and correct identification of dysphagia in patients with neurologic disease may increase quality of life and prevent or delay death. Typically, neurogenic dysphagia begins with dysphagia for liquids, but it may over time progress to include intolerance of solids.[8] Electromyography is useful in the diagnosis of oropharyngeal dysphagia in this patient subset, and it can be used to target muscles for treatment with botulinum toxin.[43]

Esophageal Motility Disorders

Musculoskeletal disorders that affect normal peristalsis may lead to dysphagia. Achalasia is the most clinically relevant degenerative disorder. In achalasia, denervation of esophageal smooth muscle over the course of many years results in progressive loss of inhibitory neurons, impairing relaxation of the lower esophagus.[44] Hypercontractile (jackhammer) esophagus and distal esophageal spasm are rare and most prevalent in patients 60 and older.[45] Both of these disorders are associated with forceful peristalsis and inappropriately timed distal esophageal spasm contractions.[44]

Infections

Although esophageal candidiasis affects less than 5% of the general population, it is the most common cause of infectious esophagitis contributing to dysphagia.[46] Risk factors for esophageal candidiasis include concomitant immunocompromising conditions, chronic proton pump inhibitor use, and tobacco use.[46] Many patients will report painful swallowing with this condition though demonstration of white, adherent mucosal plaques on endoscopy is the gold standard for diagnosis.[46] A 2 to 3 week course of antifungal medicine will typically result in resolution of this condition.[46]

Dysphagia has also been reported as a consequence of coronavirus disease 2019 (COVID-19) infection due to a post-infectious neuropathy of the cranial nerves.[47] Hospitalized patients developing such dysphagia have been shown to have reduced 6-month survival compared to those who do not develop swallowing difficulties.[48]

Systemic Sclerosis

Systemic sclerosis commonly presents with esophageal involvement resulting in dysfunction and dysphagia.[49] Difficulty with mastication, esophageal obstruction, poor esophageal motility, increased incidence of reflux, and decreased saliva production all exacerbate the dysphagia symptoms.[49] A comprehensive treatment plan aimed at addressing all factors contributing to symptoms will provide patients with the best symptom control and quality of life.[49]

Pediatric Concerns

While many of the conditions contributing to dysphagia impact older adults, physicians should remember that dysphagia may be a presenting sign of congenital neurologic diseases in infants.[50] Prematurity, respiratory and cardiac disorders, structural abnormalities such as cleft lip or palate, neuromuscular conditions as well as fetal alcohol syndrome and neonatal abstinence syndrome have all been noted to have dysphagia as a feature.[51] Typically, children will present with prolonged feeding time, food refusal, failure to thrive, coughing with meals, or increased work of breathing.[52] Although no validated screening questionnaires exist for dysphagia in children, involving a multi-disciplinary team including speech language pathologists early in the assessment of feeding difficulties can be helpful to design an individualized workup and plan of care for a child.[52]

Hospitalized Patients

Almost half of elderly patients who are hospitalized will develop some degree of oropharyngeal dysphagia.[53] Age greater than 65 years, emergent admission, need for mechanical ventilation or tracheal intubation, baseline neurologic disease, history of congestive heart failure, sepsis, or hypercholesterolemia all increase the risk of patients in the intensive care unit developing dysphagia.[54–56] Standardized algorithms for screening, assessment, and treatment of dysphagia in hospitalized patients may improve outcomes.[57] Algorithms often begin with assessment of alertness and respiratory stability followed by a swallow screen using a water swallow or multiconsistency test.[57] If unable to pass a swallow screen, a clinical swallowing evaluation by a dysphagia specialist, including a cough reflex test is indicated.[57] Alternatives for a comprehensive swallowing evaluation could include flexible endoscopic evaluation of swallowing or a videofluoroscopic swallowing study.[57]

SUMMARY

Dysphagia is a symptom of an underlying pathology rather than a disease unto itself. A thorough history and physical examination can provide rich detail that enhances a physician's ability to accurately diagnose the cause of swallowing impairment. Additional workup with EGD provides confirmation of diagnoses and may allow for treatment. Ultimately, patients benefit from treatment directed at the underlying illness targeting either cure or palliation as appropriate.

CLINICS CARE POINTS

- Dysphagia is a symptom of an underlying pathology, not a disease unto itself; thus, focusing on identifying and treating the underlying cause of dysphagia is the key.
- Opioid-induced dysphagia is an emerging concern and should be considered a risk for long-term opiate therapy.
- Dysphagia evaluations and dietary interventions lack standardization across institutions and geographic regions making ongoing research difficult.
- COVID-19-associated dysphagia may predict a worse outcome of acute infection.
- Dysphagia symptoms in children may be a first indicator of congenital neurologic disease.

DISCLOSURE

The authors have nothing to disclose.

REFERENCES

1. McCarty EB, Chao TN. Dysphagia and swallowing disorders. Med Clin North Am 2021;105(5):939–54.
2. Adkins C, Takakura W, Spiegel BMR, et al. Prevalence and characteristics of dysphagia based on a population-based survey. Clin Gastroenterol Hepatol 2020;18(9):1970–9.e2.
3. Ekberg O, Hamdy S, Woisard V, et al. Social and psychological burden of dysphagia: its impact on diagnosis and treatment. Dysphagia. Spring 2002; 17(2):139–46.
4. Wilkinson JM, Codipilly DC, Wilfahrt RP. Dysphagia: evaluation and collaborative management. Am Fam Physician 2021;103(2):97–106.
5. Bhattacharyya N. The prevalence of dysphagia among adults in the United States. Otolaryngol Head Neck Surg 2014;151(5):765–9.
6. Patel DA, Krishnaswami S, Steger E, et al. Economic and survival burden of dysphagia among inpatients in the United States. Dis Esophagus 2018 31(1):1–7.
7. Cabre M, Serra-Prat M, Palomera E, et al. Prevalence and prognostic implications of dysphagia in elderly patients with pneumonia. Age Ageing 2010;39(1):39–45.
8. Panebianco M, Marchese-Ragona R, Masiero S, et al. Dysphagia in neurological diseases: a literature review. Neurol Sci 2020;41(11):3067–73.
9. Christmas C, Rogus-Pulia N. Swallowing disorders in the older population. J Am Geriatr Soc 2019;67(12):2643–9. Epub 2019 Aug 20.
10. Lang IM. Brain stem control of the phases of swallowing. Dysphagia 2009;24(3): 333–48.
11. Cho SY, Choung RS, Saito YA, et al. Prevalence and risk factors for dysphagia: a USA community study. Neuro Gastroenterol Motil 2015;27(2):212–9.

12. Traynor BJ, Codd MB, Corr B, et al. Clinical features of amyotrophic lateral scle-rosis according to the El Escorial and Airlie House diagnostic criteria: a population-based study. Arch Neurol 2000;57(8):1171–6.
13. Scherer K, Bedlack RS, Simel DL. Does this patient have myasthenia gravis? JAMA 2005;293(15):1906–14.
14. Lee BE, Kim GH. Globus pharyngeus: a review of its etiology, diagnosis and treat-ment. World J Gastroenterol 2012;18(20):2462–71.
15. Ashraf HH, Palmer J, Dalton HR, et al. Can patients determine the level of their dysphagia? World J Gastroenterol 2017;23(6):1038–43.
16. Roeder BE, Murray JA, Dierkhising RA. Patient localization of esophageal dysphagia. Dig Dis Sci 2004;49(4):697–701.
17. Cook IJ. Diagnostic evaluation of dysphagia. Nat Clin Pract Gastroenterol Hepa-tol 2008;5(7):393–403.
18. Johnston BT. Oesophageal dysphagia: a stepwise approach to diagnosis and management. Lancet Gastroenterol Hepatol 2017;2(8):604–9.
19. Ford AC, Luthra P, Tack J, et al. Efficacy of psychotropic drugs in functional dyspepsia: systematic review and meta-analysis. Gut 2017;66(3):411–20.
20. Snyder DL, Vela MF. Opioid-induced esophageal dysfunction. Curr Opin Gastro-enterol 2020;36(4):344–50.
21. Triggs J, Pandolfino J. Recent advances in dysphagia management. F1000Res 2019;8. F1000 Faculty Rev-1527.
22. O'Horo JC, Rogus-Pulia N, Garcia-Arguello L, et al. Bedside diagnosis of dysphagia: a systematic review. J Hosp Med 2015;10(4):256–65.
23. Virvidaki IE, Nasios G, Kosmidou M, et al. Swallowing and aspiration risk: a crit-ical review of non instrumental bedside screening tests. J Clin Neurol 2018;14(3):265–74.
24. Spieker MR. Evaluating dysphagia. Am Fam Physician 2000;61(12):3639–48.
25. Varadarajulu S, Eloubeidi MA, Patel RS, et al. The yield and the predictors of esophageal pathology when upper endoscopy is used for the initial evaluation of dysphagia. Gastrointest Endosc 2005;61(7):804–8.
26. Levine B, Nielsen EW. The justifications and controversies of panendoscopy–a re-view. Ear Nose Throat J 1992;71(8):335–40, 343.
27. Hazelwood RJ, Armeson KE, Hill EG, et al. Identification of swallowing tasks from a modified barium swallow study that optimize the detection of physiological impairment. J Speech Lang Hear Res 2017;60(7):1855–63.
28. Ende F, Ickenstein GW. Respiratory and nutritional complications in oropharyn-geal dysphagia. J Gastroenterol Hepatol Res 2014;3(10):1307–12.
29. Carnaby G, Hankey GJ, Pizzi J. Behavioural intervention for dysphagia in acute stroke: a randomised controlled trial. Lancet Neurol 2006;5(1):31–7.
30. Perez I, Smithard DG, Davies H. Pharmacological treatment of dysphagia in stroke. Dysphagia 1998;13:12–6.
31. Knigge MA, Thibeault SL. Swallowing outcomes after cricopharyngeal myotomy: a systematic review. Head Neck 2018;40(1):203–12.
32. Krekeler BN, Broadfoot CK, Johnson S, et al. Patient adherence to dysphagia recommendations: a systematic review. Dysphagia 2018;33(2):173–84. Erratum in: Dysphagia. 2018 May 4.
33. Cichero JA, Lam P, Steele CM, et al. Development of international terminology and definitions for texture-modified foods and thickened fluids used in dysphagia management: the IDDSI framework. Dysphagia 2017;32(2):293–314.
34. Peñalva-Arigita A, Lecha M, Sansano A, et al. Adherence to commercial food thickener in patients with oropharyngeal dysphagia. BMC Geriatr 2024;24(1):67.

35. Committee ASoP, Pasha SF, Acosta RD, et al. The role of endoscopy in the evaluation and management of dysphagia. Gastrointest Endosc 2014;79(2):191–201.
36. Vakil N, Moayyedi P, Fennerty MB, et al. Limited value of alarm features in the diagnosis of upper gastrointestinal malignancy: systematic review and meta-analysis. Gastroenterology 2006;131(2):390–401.
37. Moayyedi P, Lacy BE, Andrews CN, et al. ACG and CAG clinical guideline: management of dyspepsia. Am J Gastroenterol 2017;112(7):988–1013 [published correction appears in *Am J Gastroenterol*. 2017;112(9):1484].
38. Richter JE, Rubenstein JH. Presentation and epidemiology of gastroesophageal reflux disease. Gastroenterology 2018;154(2):267–76.
39. Lenz CJ, Leggett C, Katzka DA, et al. Food impaction: etiology over 35 years and association with eosinophilic esophagitis. Dis Esophagus 2019;32(4):pii.
40. Dellon ES, Katzka DA, Collins MH, et al. MP-101-06 Investigators. Budesonide oral suspension improves symptomatic, endoscopic, and histologic parameters compared with placebo in patients with eosinophilic esophagitis. Gastroenterology 2017;152(4):776–86.e5.
41. Lucendo AJ, Arias Á, González-Cervera J, et al. Empiric 6-food elimination diet induced and maintained prolonged remission in patients with adult eosinophilic esophagitis: a prospective study on the food cause of the disease. J Allergy Clin Immunol 2013;131(3):797–804.
42. Robbins J. The evolution of swallowing neuroanatomy and physiology in humans: a practical perspective. Ann Neurol 1999;46:279–80.
43. Restivo DA, Marchese-Ragona R, Lauria G, et al. Botulinum toxin treatment for oropharyngeal dysphagia associated with diabetic neuropathy. Diabetes Care 2006;29(12):2650–3.
44. Wilkinson JM, Halland M. Esophageal motility disorders. Am Fam Physician 2020; 102(5):291–6.
45. Pandolfino JE, Roman S, Carlson D, et al. Distal esophageal spasm in high-resolution esophageal pressure topography: defining clinical phenotypes. Gastroenterology 2011;141(2):469–75.
46. Mohamed AA, Lu XL, Mounmin FA. Diagnosis and treatment of esophageal candidiasis: current updates. Chin J Gastroenterol Hepatol 2019;2019:3585136.
47. Cavalagl A, Peiti G, Conti C, et al. Cranial nerves: impairment in post-acute oropharyngeal dysphagia after COVID-19. Eur J Phys Rehabil Med 2020;56: 853–7.
48. Martin-Martinez A, Ortega O, Viñas P, et al. COVID-19 is associated with oropharyngeal dysphagia and malnutrition in hospitalized patients during the spring 2020 wave of the pandemic. Clin Nutr 2022;41(12):2996–3006.
49. Kadakuntla A, Juneja A, Sattler S, et al. Dysphagia, reflux and related sequelae due to altered physiology in scleroderma. World J Gastroenterol 2021;27(31): 5201–18.
50. Abadie V, Couly G. Congenital feeding and swallowing disorders. Handb Clin Neurol 2013;113:1539–49.
51. Dodrill P, Gosa MM. Pediatric dysphagia: physiology, assessment, and management. Ann Nutr Metab 2015;66(Suppl 5):24–31.
52. Lawlor CM, Choi S. Diagnosis and management of pediatric dysphagia: a review. JAMA Otolaryngol Head Neck Surg 2020;146(2):183–91.
53. Clave P, Rofes L, Carrion S, et al. Pathophysiology, relevance and natural history of oropharyngeal dysphagia among older people. Nestle Nutr Inst Workshop Ser 2012;72:57–66.

54. Zuercher P, Schenk NV, Moret C, et al. Risk factors for dysphagia in ICU patients after invasive mechanical ventilation. Chest 2020;158(5):1983–91.
55. Xia C, Ji J. The characteristics and predicators of post-extubation dysphagia in ICU patients with endotracheal intubationDysphagia 2023;38(1):253–9.
56. Skoretz SA, Flowers H, Martino R. The incidence of dysphagia following intubation: a systematic reviewChest 2010;137(3):665–73.
57. Likar R, Aroyo I, Bangert K, et al. Management of swallowing disorders in ICU patients - a multinational expert opinion. J Crit Care 2024;79:154447.

Moving?

Make sure your subscription moves with you!

To notify us of your new address, find your **Clinics Account Number** (located on your mailing label above your name), and contact customer service at:

Email: journalscustomerservice-usa@elsevier.com

800-654-2452 (subscribers in the U.S. & Canada)
314-447-8871 (subscribers outside of the U.S. & Canada)

Fax number: 314-447-8029

Elsevier Health Sciences Division
Subscription Customer Service
3251 Riverport Lane
Maryland Heights, MO 63043

*To ensure uninterrupted delivery of your subscription, please notify us at least 4 weeks in advance of move.

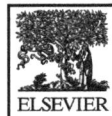

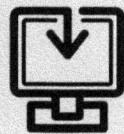

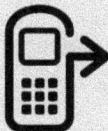

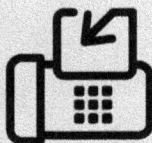

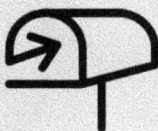

ELSEVIER